Daily DASH for Weight Loss

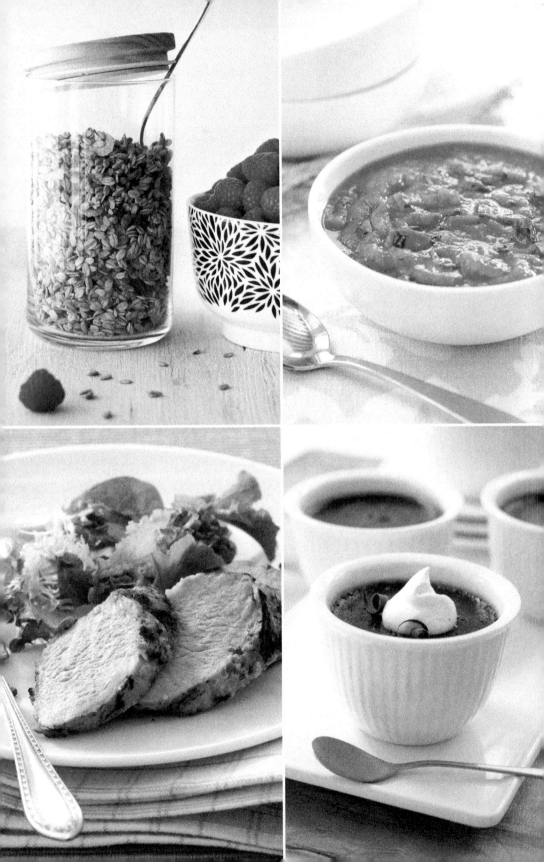

DAILY DASH

— FOR —

WEIGHT LOSS

A Day-By-Day
DASH Diet
Weight Loss Plan

**ROCKRIDGE
PRESS**

Contents

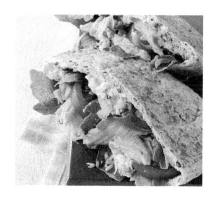

PART ONE

—————————

The DASH Diet

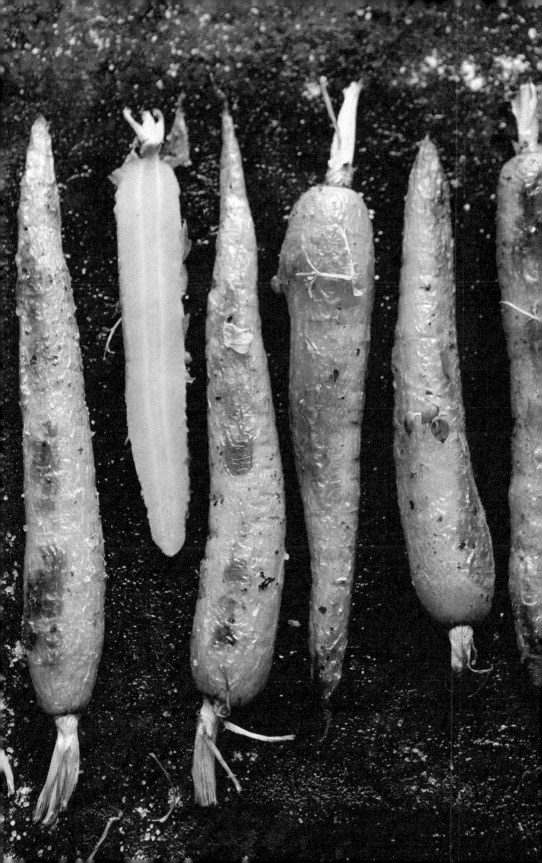

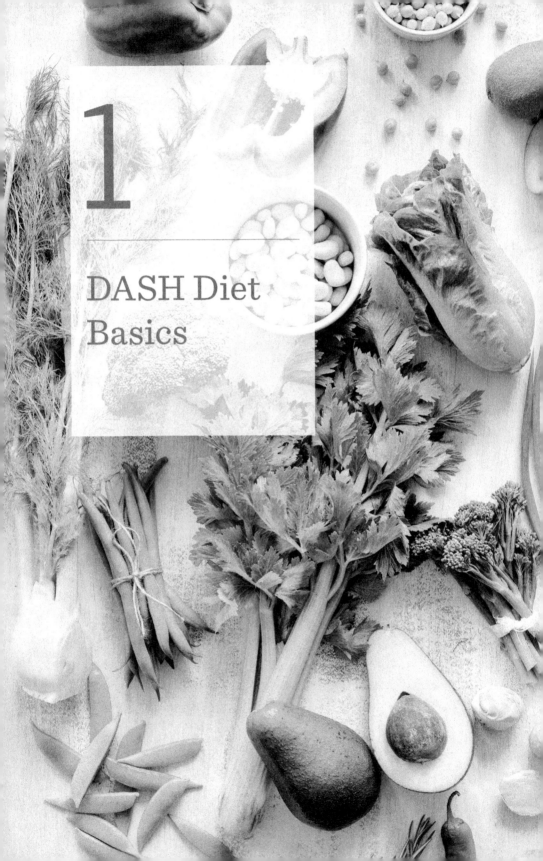

1

DASH Diet Basics

WHAT IS THE DASH DIET?

Losing weight and reducing blood pressure are two goals with a common solution: the DASH diet. The Dietary Approaches to Stop Hypertension (DASH) plan was developed for people who have to manage high blood pressure (also known as hypertension). It is an eating system, not a short-term fix, and it will help you lose weight and reduce your blood pressure.

The DASH dietary program is a remarkably beneficial tool for weight reduction. The ongoing research on hypertension has linked high blood pressure not only to what you eat, but also to body weight. If you are overweight, your heart must work harder than normal to move blood into the extra tissues. Though up to 60 percent of people diagnosed with hypertension are considered obese, the other 40 percent are not obese but are, to some degree, over their ideal weight. The risk of hypertension doubles if your body weight is just 20 percent above your ideal weight, but reducing your weight by as little as 5 or 10 percent has a positive impact on blood pressure.

The number one thing you can do to improve your blood pressure and your overall health is to reduce your body weight. By developing dietary habits that promote long-term health and slow but steady weight loss, the DASH diet can help you lose weight and keep it off while also helping you reduce your blood pressure.

Reducing Sodium: The First Step

The link between high blood pressure and eating a high-sodium diet has been scientifically evaluated and confirmed. Studies in the United States and other countries have demonstrated that when you reduce the amount of sodium in your diet, the result is a drop in blood pressure. The American Heart Association recommends that adults consume no more than 1,500 milligrams of sodium each day, but most Americans consume as much as 2,300 milligrams of sodium per day. The effect on blood pressure of reducing the amount of sodium you eat each day is quite fast. Most people experience a drop in blood pressure within two weeks of implementing DASH, and the changes within eight weeks can be dramatic.

In addition to helping you lose weight and control blood pressure, following DASH offers other health incentives. In recent years, as a result of even more scientific testing and analysis, DASH has been shown to reduce the risk of many types of cancer, improve HDL and LDL cholesterol levels, and decrease the risk of kidney stones. Plus, there are no negative side effects associated with following DASH.

Managing your weight is a lifelong commitment and involves modifying diet, exercise, and other lifestyle habits. It's also important to eat a variety of healthy foods. The DASH dietary program, in addition to reducing sodium, incorporates a balance of foods from many food groups and boosts intake of certain minerals that support a healthy circulatory system.

HEALTH BENEFITS OF THE DASH DIET

Most people don't realize that they have high blood pressure unless they visit a physician and a measurement is taken. Hypertension usually has no noticeable symptoms, but it has a serious effect on your health. Some of the consequences of unchecked blood pressure are:

* *Arteriosclerosis, or hardening of the arteries.* Hypertension stiffens the arterial walls, which leads to a cascade of negative effects. These include an accelerated buildup of cholesterol and fat in the blood vessels and a slower flow of blood through the body, which in turn increases risk of heart attack and stroke.

◆ *Heart attack.* When the arteries cannot properly perform their job of moving oxygenated blood from the heart to the body's tissues and back, the heart muscle does not receive enough oxygen. If the flow of blood stops, even for a short time, the heart muscle suffers irreversible damage. Chest pain from reduced blood flow (angina) can also occur.

◆ *Stroke.* Reduced blood flow as a result of a narrowing of the blood vessels to the brain can cause permanent damage to the brain. If there is a blockage in one of the arteries, a stroke can occur. Stroke can also be the result of high blood pressure causing a break in a weakened blood vessel in the brain.

◆ *Enlarged heart.* The extra work being done by the heart when it is working at high pressure can cause the heart muscle to thicken and stretch. Over time, the heart no longer functions properly, causing a buildup of fluid in the lungs (congestive heart failure).

◆ *Kidney damage.* When blood flow to the kidneys is restricted, the kidneys function less effectively. When the kidneys filter less fluid and waste, these substances can build up in the blood or the kidneys may fail altogether.

These conditions can be prevented by managing blood pressure. By changing your diet to DASH, you can experience these benefits in as little as two weeks.

A few of the benefits of the DASH dietary program are:

◆ Lower blood pressure, both systolic (the pressure that blood exerts on the artery walls when the heart beats) and diastolic (the pressure that blood exerts on the artery walls when the heart rests between beats) measurements

◆ Lower blood cholesterol levels

- Lower homocysteine levels (a naturally occurring amino acid in the blood plasma, found to increase the risk of heart disease, stroke, Alzheimer's disease, and osteoporosis)
- Reduced risk of cancer
- Reduced risk of osteoporosis
- An improved quality of life
- An improved sense of well-being

DASH AND THE MODERN DIET

It is no coincidence that the rise of hypertension in the past quarter century has occurred simultaneously with a decline in our consumption of whole grains, fruits, and vegetables and an increase in our consumption of sodium, sugar, and fat. The DASH diet seeks to reduce your intake of sodium, sugar, and less healthful fats and boost your intake of whole grains, fruits, vegetables, and healthful fats. By increasing the amounts of whole foods you eat, the nutrients—vitamins, minerals, and antioxidants—your body needs to function well will also increase and the negative effects of a diet high in refined and highly processed foods will decrease.

A clinical study from 1997 that involved hundreds of people with high blood pressure looked at the effects of diet on blood pressure. Over an eight-week period, study participants were asked to follow one of three dietary programs:

1. A modern American diet, but with more fruits and vegetables
2. The DASH diet, or one high in fruits, vegetables, and low-fat dairy products but with less red meat and less sugar-added foods and drinks
3. A modern American diet, low in fruits, vegetables, and low-fat dairy products

The DASH diet lowered systolic and diastolic blood pressure the most. The American diet that was high in fruits and vegetables also lowered blood pressure, but not as much as DASH. These results are roughly equivalent to the results from using blood-pressure medicines. The people in the study group experienced these changes within two weeks of modifying their diets.

The human body has not changed much in millenia. What has changed in the last fifty years is the kind of foods we eat. Convenience foods and many packaged foods use salt as a preservative and for flavor. Placing a salt shaker on the table when we sit down to eat is customary for most people. We do it without thinking, just as we shake salt onto our food before even tasting it. Our bodies need some salt for optimum function, so DASH does not seek to eliminate salt entirely, just to reduce it.

THE DASH DIETARY PROGRAM

The DASH dietary program is a balanced one that incorporates foods from all food groups, including proteins, carbohydrates, and fats. Your body needs all of these for optimum performance and health. DASH does not eliminate any foods, but does emphasize specific types of proteins, carbohydrates, and fats that help you lose weight, lower your blood pressure, and improve your overall health.

DASH includes daily portions of:

* Whole grains, such as rice, pasta, and cereal

* Whole fruits, such as apricots, mangoes, and apples

* Whole vegetables, such as asparagus, peas, broccoli, and squash

* Low-fat dairy products, such as low-fat yogurt, milk, and cheese

* Lean proteins, such as poultry and certain cuts of lamb and pork

* Fish and seafood, such as salmon and shrimp

+ Nuts and seeds, such as sesame seeds, almonds, and cashews

+ Legumes, such as chickpeas and black beans

+ Oils, such as olive and canola

These items are permitted in small amounts:

+ Processed meats, such as deli meat

+ Chips, crackers, and energy bars

+ Sugar-sweetened beverages, such as soda and fruit juice

+ Cakes, cookies, and other bakery items

Proteins: Go Lean

Proteins enable our bodies to do countless things, like grow and replace tissues, and build and maintain muscles. Any diet need to include a healthy amount of protein, and proteins are often at the center of weight-loss diets because they're satisfying and help combat water retention. With DASH, slow, steady weight loss is the goal. Eating protein is part of the DASH dietary program, but DASH also seeks to add lower-fat sources of whole protein to your eating plan. Low-fat animal proteins, seafood, and vegetarian proteins are included in DASH.

Keep in mind, too, that our bodies need some cholesterol—we use it to make hormones—but too much can have negative consequences. Found mostly in animal products, such as meat, egg yolks, and milk, cholesterol is also found in some seafood and fish. DASH strives for a balance of proteins from animals, seafood, and plants. Lower-fat proteins, such as reduced fat dairy, egg whites, and meats sourced from the leaner cuts of animals, are included in DASH.

Carbohydrates: Choose Slow Carbs

Carbohydrates are an important source of fuel for the body. Your brain, in particular, likes having a ready source of fuel, which it receives from digested carbohydrates. Quality carbohydrates, those that release glucose in a slow, steady manner and not in a sudden, big rush, are part of the balanced DASH dietary system. These "slow carbs" have a steadying effect on blood sugar and insulin. They contain enough fiber that your body must work harder to digest them. For instance, whole grains are minimally processed and contain all parts of the kernel—the germ, bran, and endosperm. Seek out grains where the germ, bran, and endosperm have never been removed, altered, or processed.

Whole wheat, long thought to be a slow carb, is just the opposite. Gram for gram, modern wheat increases blood sugar to a greater degree than other carbohydrates such as garbanzo beans or potato chips. The type of wheat you choose can have a significant impact on your wellness and your ability to lose weight. While DASH does not entirely eliminate wheat, it is prudent to reduce the amount of wheat in your diet. Choose carbohydrates that are made from gluten-free grains such as quinoa and brown rice, or unadulterated forms of wheat such as whole spelt or farro, wheat's ancient cousins that do not increase blood sugar as modern whole wheat does. Limit foods made from modern wheat strains.

Fats: The Good, the Bad, and the Really Bad

All humans need fats for optimum health. Our bodies use fats for countless functions, including for energy and the protection of nerve cells, and to turn genes on and off and regulate inflammation.

Fat gets a bad rap. The negative health consequences associated with fat only apply to certain types. For instance, saturated fats (found mostly in meat and dairy products) and trans fats (man-made fats, present in partially hydrogenated oils) increase cholesterol levels, which can cause major circulatory problems and related health issues. These are discussed at length in the list that follows.

When attempting to lose weight and reduce blood pressure with DASH, you need to eat more healthful fats and fewer unhealthy fats, and select low-fat options when eating dairy products. To help you lose weight and lower your cholesterol, DASH is low in total fat and in saturated fat. This is consistent with recommendations from the American Heart Association.

There are a few key terms that come up frequently in any discussion about dietary fats and which ones to eat. Here is what you need to know:

+ **Cholesterol** is a type of fat found in the blood and some foods. Cholesterol is used by your body to make some hormones and build cells, so it is important to eat some cholesterol. However, too much cholesterol in the blood has negative health implications.

+ **HDL**, high-density lipoproteins, carry cholesterol from the body's tissues to the liver for excretion. Because HDLs move cholesterol out of arteries and keep cholesterol from building up, they are often referred to as "good" cholesterol.

+ **LDL**, or low-density lipoproteins, carry cholesterol to the body's tissues. LDLs are the main source of cholesterol buildup and blockage in the arteries. Because high LDL levels are a risk factor for heart disease and other cardiovascular problems, LDLs are referred to as "bad" cholesterol.

+ **Triglycerides**, like cholesterol, are a type of fat found in the blood. When you eat, your body converts any extra calories into stored energy and places it in fat cells for later use. High triglycerides are also a risk factor for heart disease.

+ **Unsaturated fats** are essential for optimum wellness. They lower LDL cholesterol but do not lower HDL cholesterol. They guard against heart attack and stroke, and help control blood sugar and inflammation. Unsaturated fats are sources of omega-3 and omega-6 fatty acids, which reduce the risk of heart, brain, and liver disorders, among other benefits. Good sources of unsaturated fats include salmon and almonds.

* *Monounsaturated fat* is a type of unsaturated fat that is liquid at room temperature. It lowers LDL cholesterol and boosts HDL cholesterol. These fats also ease inflammation and improve the body's sensitivity to insulin. Olive oil is a good source of mono-unsaturated fats.

* *Polyunsaturated fat*, an unsaturated fat, is also liquid at room temperature and is found in most vegetable oils. This fat provides healthful omega-3 and omega-6 fatty acids. Like mono-unsaturated fats, polyunsaturated fats lower LDL cholesterol and boost HDL cholesterol. They provide the body with count-less other benefits.

* *Saturated fats* come mostly from animal products and are linked to heart and circulatory disease, insulin resistance, and other health problems. The DASH dietary program includes some saturated fats to support optimum health, in foods like low-fat dairy products. By eating low-fat dairy products, you can boost calcium intake while avoiding the added calories and fat of whole-fat dairy products.

* *Trans-fatty acids* are found in small amounts in various ani-mal products such as beef, pork, lamb, butter, and milk. TFAs are also formed during the process of hydrogenation. They increase harmful LDL and decrease protective HDL.

In packaged foods and fast food, TFAs offer a shelf-stable source of fat. Once the food labels on packaged foods—the little box titled "Nutrition Facts"—were required to list TFAs, many manufacturers removed some or all of the TFAs from their products. In most cases, the TFAs were replaced with saturated fat. Read labels carefully on all packaged foods, including crackers, bread, and baked goods, as these products are often a hidden source of saturated fat.

Eating out can be a minefield of foods loaded with saturated fats and trans-fatty acids. Many restaurants, especially but not exclusively fast-food chains, still use trans fats in the form of partially hydrogenated oil to make fried foods.

The DASH eating program does not include any TFAs. These fats should be avoided to lose weight and lower blood pressure.

Eat Your Minerals: Potassium, Calcium, and Magnesium

You already knew that calcium is important for the health of your bones and teeth. Calcium is also important for heart health. In a series of studies, low-fat dairy products were found to play an important role in reducing the risk of hypertension, diabetes, and cardiovascular problems. Calcium by itself is not enough to lower blood pressure, but it does help relax the arteries and encourages the body to eliminate sodium. Dairy products in particular appear to contain additional nutrients that work in conjunction with calcium to lower blood pressure. Most Americans do not get enough calcium in their diets to achieve these benefits. DASH includes plenty of low-fat dairy and other sources of calcium.

A study from the early 1990s proved that increasing your potassium intake, equal to three servings of fruits or vegetables each day, directly correlates to a reduction in blood pressure. Potassium is a "vasodilator," meaning it relaxes the muscle cells that make up the walls of blood vessels. It does a job similar to blood pressure medicines, which are also vasodilators. Potassium also helps the body get rid of sodium through the urine. The DASH plan incorporates lots of the potassium-rich foods you need to eat to achieve these benefits.

Magnesium affects blood pressure in a few different ways. Like potassium, it is a vasodilator that controls the access of calcium to arterial cells. Low levels of magnesium are associated with the increased activity of an enzyme that contributes to hypertension. Magnesium also helps promote proper cell function by maintaining the proper ratio of calcium, potassium, and sodium, both within and outside cells. As with calcium and potassium, most Americans do not get enough magnesium. Following DASH ensures that you do.

A Word About Alcohol

Regular consumption of a glass of red wine or two each day has been positively linked to improved circulation and heart health. Red wine has been demonstrated to boost HDL and reduce arterio-sclerosis. Drinking one or two drinks of any type each day does not increase blood pressure. However, more than two drinks each day has been shown to have the opposite effect. In fact, independent of all factors that lead to hypertension, consumption of more than three drinks a day on a continued basis can cause hypertension and lead to hemorrhagic stroke.

FOODS TO ENJOY

Whole, minimally processed vegetables and fruits are all smart DASH choices and should be eaten at every meal and snack. To boost your intake of potassium, magnesium, and calcium from sources other than dairy, you may select from a huge range of fiber-rich options. Eating foods from the following lists is a keystone of DASH.

Sources of calcium

Almonds

Blackstrap molasses

Calcium-fortified cereals

Calcium-fortified low-fat soy milk and almond milk

Calcium-fortified orange juice

Calcium-fortified tofu

Canned salmon and sardines

Dark green leafy vegetables such as collard greens, kale, turnips, spinach, bok choy, and broccoli

Figs, both fresh and dried (but especially dried)

Low-fat dairy such as plain yogurt, milk, and cheese

Navy beans, chickpeas, and other legumes

Sesame seeds

Sources of potassium

Apricots, especially dried apricots

Asparagus

Avocados

Bananas

Cantaloupe and honeydew melon

Milk and yogurt

Navy beans, chickpeas, and other legumes

Pears

Potatoes and sweet potatoes

Pumpkins and other squashes, such as butternut and acorn

Sources of magnesium

Avocados

Black beans, black-eyed peas, and other legumes

Cocoa

Dark green leafy vegetables such as collard greens, kale, turnips, spinach, bok choy, and broccoli

Fatty fish such as halibut and mackerel

Magnesium-fortified breakfast cereal

Nuts, including almonds, walnuts, cashews, and pistachios

Quinoa

Seeds, including sesame and pumpkin

Whole grains such as brown rice and millet

Sources of smart fats

Fatty fish such as wild salmon, herring, sardines, and halibut

Low-fat yogurt, low-fat milk, evaporated skim milk, part-skim
ricotta, light sour cream

Nuts and seeds such as walnuts, almonds, cashews, flaxseed, hemp
seeds, pumpkin seeds, pine nuts, and pistachios

Oils such as olive, canola, flaxseed, hemp, pumpkin seed, and
grape seed

Sources of smart proteins

Fish such as salmon, herring, and mackerel

Lean meats, including buffalo, leaner cuts of grass-fed beef, lamb,
pork, and skinless chicken and turkey

Legumes such as black-eyed peas, beans of any kind (black, white,
navy, pinto), soybeans, lentils, and carob

Low-fat dairy products

Nuts such as walnuts, pistachios, almonds, pine nuts, and pecans

Shellfish, including crab, mussels, oysters, and shrimp

Sources of smart carbohydrates

Brown and wild rice

Bulgur, barley, spelt, farro, and other forms of ancient grains

Legumes such as black-eyed peas, beans of any kind (black, white,
navy, pinto), soybeans, lentils, and carob

Popcorn

Whole or flaked quinoa

Whole or rolled oats

FOODS TO AVOID

The items listed here are high in salt and, in general, should not be eaten regularly. You may eat these foods occasionally, but they should not be a regular part of your diet. If you cannot eliminate these items, look for versions that contain no added salt or lower salt.

Condiments such as ketchup, mustard, and mayonnaise

Crackers and baked goods

Deep-fried foods

Instant mixes like instant soup or breading mixes for
    chicken and pork

Margarine

Packaged soup

Pasta dishes

Pizza

Premade salad dressing

Snack foods such as potato chips and pretzels

Soy sauce

Whole-fat cheese

TEN REASONS WHY THE DASH DIET TRULY WORKS FOR WEIGHT LOSS

Although the DASH diet was not originally designed for weight loss, followers of the DASH plan have quickly discovered that the particular combination of foods and nutrients in the program lead to reduced blood pressure, improved weight loss, and enhanced over-all health. Specific reasons include:

1. The DASH diet focuses on whole natural foods, including plenty of fresh vegetables and fruits. It is well known that plant-based diets support weight loss and general good health. But many people do not include the recommended number of servings of these nutrient-packed foods in their daily diet. This means that they are instead probably eating food that contains more calories and fat, which can lead to weight gain. Simply following DASH diet guidelines will ensure that you fill up on low-calorie, nutrient-rich vegetables and fruit instead of fattening food choices.

2. You will eat fewer calories. The simplified formula for weight loss is that if you eat fewer calories than you expend, you will lose weight. The DASH diet is built on lower-calorie foods because you are not eating much sugar, saturated fat, or empty processed food calories. This equals fewer calories on your plate and eventual weight loss.

3. You will eat real food, not shakes, bars, or pills. Sitting at a table full of friends and family who are enjoying a good meal while you slurp a weight-loss shake is not motivating and could be downright depressing. The DASH diet contains normal food and allows you to make choices that do not leave you feeling deprived or singled out.

4. DASH does not have lists of eating rules to follow. Many weight-loss diets do not take into account the difficulties people can encounter trying to fit their unique lives and needs into dieting rules. This usually creates a situation where people fall off the diet and gain their weight back. DASH is flexible and provides common-sense guidelines for all situations you might encounter, like eating out, events, busy schedules, and traveling.

5. DASH is not a fad diet. It is not a short-term quick-fix eating plan, but rather a long-term, sensible, satisfying lifestyle change designed to produce sustainable weight loss and to lower blood pressure. And because you adopt the eating program for life, you experience no rebound weight gain.

6. You will not be hungry. Whole natural foods are filling and feature ingredients low on the glycemic index. This means your body digests them more slowly and you feel full longer. You could eat a small bag of French fries that might equal a cup of food or you can enjoy an entire plate of a colorful tossed salad and a piece of grilled chicken for the same calorie amount. Which will keep you full longer and eliminate a binge-eating compulsion?

7. Processed foods are eliminated. The DASH diet consists of foods that are natural and unprocessed. Processed foods have been linked conclusively with weight gain, so removing these products can increase weight-loss potential and improve health.

8. Exercise is an important component of DASH. Although the right food choices are the foundation of this diet plan, it is also recommended that you work out a minimum of five times per week with a variety of activities that cover cardio, strength training, and flexibility. Exercise also supports and accelerates weight-loss goals.

9. The DASH diet includes all food groups. Many weight-loss diets are geared around excluding certain food groups or ingredients, which can make them difficult to follow. The DASH diet incorporates all types of food, even healthy fat, because the body needs a wide array of nutrients to function well. This all-encompassing eating style makes following DASH easy and weight loss within reach.

10. You can eat an occasional treat. People can feel deprived pretty quickly when dieting, and this is usually the primary reason dieters quit a particular plan. Having permission to have a piece of chocolate, a cookie, or a glass of wine can alleviate those cravings and the feeling of being deprived. This means that you can stick to the DASH diet and lose the weight.

2

Losing Weight with the DASH Diet

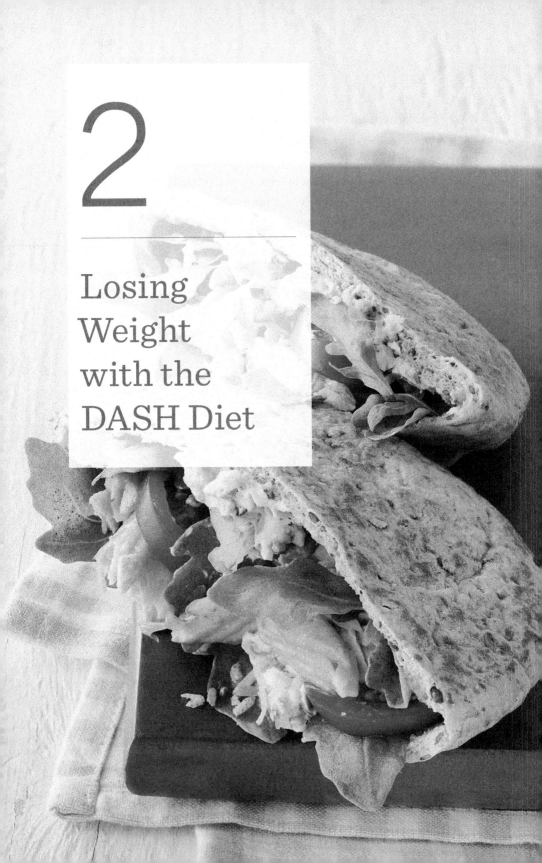

HOW THE DASH DIET HELPS WITH WEIGHT LOSS

DASH is a way of eating that will help you lose weight and reduce high blood pressure. Learning how to eat for weight loss and to reduce blood pressure is easy. DASH looks at portion size and the number of portions of each of the food groups you should eat each day. That's it.

Almost any food can fit into DASH if it is portioned appropriately. Even foods that are not healthful, such as the list of foods to avoid, can occasionally be included. The key is to remember that these foods should not be eaten frequently and, if you do eat them, do so only in small amounts.

Be sure to eat a balance of proteins, carbohydrates, and fats at each meal to help you feel satisfied and full. By eating in balance and eating a majority of the foods recommended each day, your portions will resume the appropriate size for your caloric needs.

DASH works because you feel full after each meal and snack. A day's worth of calories includes lots of slow-to-digest fiber in the form of whole carbohydrates, fats, and proteins to keep you feeling full longer. Hunger is kept at bay. When you are not hungry as often, you eat less. When you eat less, you consume fewer calories. When you consume fewer calories, you lose weight.

You can lose weight on any kind of diet, and you can gain weight on any kind of diet. The key is not to consume more calories than your body needs each day. Exercise is an important tool for weight loss and managing a healthy weight. By adding exercise, it is possible to lose weight without reducing calories. Of course, reducing calories and exercising regularly is the best, most healthful combination and is recommended for everyone following the DASH plan..

To lose weight safely, setting realistic goals is the first step. Healthy weight loss means losing no more than one to two pounds a week. Losing weight at this slow but steady pace comes with an incentive: most people who lose weight using the slow but steady approach keep the weight off and maintain their new, healthier lifestyle. The American Heart Association recommends that those beginning a weight-loss regimen aim for a reduction of 10 percent of body weight as a starting goal.

To get started, most people need to eat about 500 calories a day less than they ate before. By eating 500 calories a day less than you burn, you can lose that one to two pounds of body fat each week. If you eat about 2,500 calories each day, your new goal will be 2,000 calories each day. To get a handle on how to remove 500 calories from your eating regimen, let's look at two tools: DASH and number of servings, and what constitutes a serving on DASH.

DASH FOODS AND SERVING SIZES

The DASH diet is very flexible when it comes to the range of foods you can eat on the plan, but it does recommend certain portion sizes and number of servings. Healthy food can cause weight gain if you eat more calories than your body is burning. Portion size is often the calculation that creates issues with weight, because a bowlful of cereal can actually be four servings when you pour out the suggested amount for a serving indicated on the label. If you want to eat four servings of grain in the morning, that is fine, but then you need to calculate how many grain portions you can have during the rest of the day. The process of counting might seem complicated to start with, but eventually you will be a DASH veteran and able to calculate a portion size automatically just by looking at it.

DASH Foods and Serving Sizes

FOOD	PORTION SIZE
GRAIN	
Multigrain or whole grain bread	1 slice
English muffin	½ muffin
Multigrain or whole-wheat bun	1 bun
Bagel	½ bagel
Whole grain tortilla	One 6-inch tortilla
Dry cereal or grains (quinoa, barley, millet, oats, wheat berries)	1 ounce
Cooked whole-grain pasta	½ cup
Cooked brown or wild rice	½ cup
Cooked cereal	½ cup
VEGETABLES	
Raw leafy vegetables (spinach, beet greens, kale, mixed greens)	1 cup
Raw vegetables (beans, bell peppers, corn, carrots, peas, radishes, cucumbers)	½ cup
Cooked vegetables	½ cup
Frozen vegetables	½ cup
Vegetable juice	6
FRUITS	
Whole fresh fruit (apple, orange, pear, banana, peach, plum)	1 whole fruit
Melon	¼ melon
Fresh fruit (papaya, mango, grapes, berries)	½ cup
Frozen fruit	½ cup

➤

> ➤ DASH Foods and Serving Sizes

FOOD	PORTION SIZE
FRUITS *continued*	
Canned fruit	½ cup
Dried fruit	¼ cup
Fruit juice	6 ounces
DAIRY PRODUCTS	
Skim or fat-free milk	8 ounces
Skim chocolate milk	8 ounces
Fat-free yogurt	1 cup
Fat-free cottage cheese	½ cups
Cheese	1½ ounces
Egg whites	2 egg whites
Egg substitute	1
LEAN MEATS	
Lean ground beef	3 ounces
Beef, trimmed of fat	4 ounces
Lamb, trimmed of fat	4 ounces
Pork, trimmed of fat	3 ounces
Lean ground pork	4 ounces
Bison	4 ounces

DASH Foods and Serving Sizes

FOOD	PORTION SIZE
POULTRY	
Ground chicken breast	3 ounces
Chicken breast, skinless, boneless	4 ounces
Lean ground turkey breast	3 ounces
Turkey breast	4 ounces
FISH AND SHELLFISH	
Fresh fish	5 to 6 ounces
Frozen fish	5 to 6 ounces
Mussels	8 mussels
Shrimp	6 ounces
NUTS AND SEEDS	
Nut milk	8 ounces
Nuts	1 ounce
Seeds (sesame seeds, flaxseed, sunflower seeds)	1 ounce
Natural nut butters	2 tablespoons
LEGUMES	
Lentils	½ cup cooked
Black beans	½ cup cooked
Peas	½ cup cooked
Chickpeas	½ cup cooked
Navy beans	½ cup cooked

➤ DASH Foods and Serving Sizes

FOOD	PORTION SIZE
FATS AND OILS	
Olive oil	1 tablespoon
Unsalted butter	1 tablespoon
Oils (canola, walnut, sesame)	1 tablespoon
Cooking spray	As required
SWEETENERS	
Honey	1 tablespoon
Brown rice syrup	1 tablespoon
Molasses	1 tablespoon
Maple syrup	1 tablespoon
PANTRY ITEMS AND MISCELLANEOUS	
Fat-free mayonnaise	1 tablespoon
Low-sodium ketchup	1 tablespoon
Mustard	1 tablespoon
Unsweetened applesauce	½ cup
Sodium-free broth	1 cup
Tofu	4 ounces
Vinegar	2 tablespoons
Popcorn (plain)	3 cups

DASH SERVINGS PER DAY

When considering the number of portions allotted on the DASH diet per day, make sure you get a good balance of everything, especially carbohydrates (grains, vegetables, fruit) and protein, so you feel satiated after each meal. Feeling full is a hallmark of the DASH plan and a key factor in why it works for weight loss. If you are feeling satisfied and not hungry, there is less chance of food cravings, bingeing, and inappropriate food choices.

Food Groups and Serving Sizes per Day or Week

FOOD GROUP	SERVINGS PER DAY OR WEEK
Grains	7 to 8 per day
Vegetables	4 to 5 per day
Fruits	4 to 5 per day
Dairy	2 to 3 per day
Meats, poultry, and fish	2 or fewer per day
Legumes, nuts, and seeds	4 to 5 per week
Sweeteners	5 or fewer per week
Fats and oils	2 to 3 per day

One of the best strategies for making sure you are following the recommended portion sizes and total daily food amounts of the DASH diet is to keep track of your food in a journal. This record is especially informative and important when you are new to DASH, because people often eat more than they think they do during the course of the day. You will also be grateful for your food journal if your weight loss stalls, because you can simply look at what you've been eating and see where there might be room for changes. Make sure you eat the amount of calories suggested each day, because starving yourself is not a DASH strategy and can damage your health, depending on what nutrients you are not getting enough of.

THE IMPORTANCE OF EXERCISE

Regular exercise helps control blood sugar levels, fights inflammation, and can lower bad cholesterol and raise good cholesterol. Exercise is a known stress-reliever. Regular exercise can lower the arteries and makes them more supple, reducing the pressure on the artery walls.

Beyond the eating plan, the second part of this successful weight-loss program is exercise. This does not mean hours of sweat-drenched reps in the gym or running miles on the treadmill. Exercise comes in many forms suitable for your starting activity level and physical condition. Keep in mind that you should always consult your doctor before jumping into a new exercise routine, especially if you have been sedentary or in poor health.

Exercise has many benefits beyond weight loss that will help you embrace your DASH diet adventure with enthusiasm. Regular moderate exercise can:

* Improve sleep

* Increase energy

* Support weight loss

* Improve general physical health

* Boost metabolism

* Improve sex drive

* Boost your self-confidence

* Decrease rate of aging

* Improve cognitive function and mood

- Help control blood sugar levels
- Fight inflammation
- Lower bad cholesterol and raise good cholesterol
- Relieve stress
- Lower blood pressure

Scientists think that because exercise moves blood through your body more quickly than normal, it clears the arteries and makes them more supple, reducing the pressure on the artery walls. Exercise is an important tool in the DASH toolkit. As mentioned earlier, exercise can help you lose weight, which is the single most important thing you can do to lower your blood pressure. Even a small loss of weight will have beneficial impact on blood pressure as well as reducing the risk of heart disease and diabetes.

Before undertaking an exercise program, you need to know more about how the body functions.

CALORIE NEEDS FOR WEIGHT LOSS

Your body needs a certain number of calories every day to function effectively. To get this number, you have to calculate your basal metabolic rate (BMR) using your height, weight, and activity level. The following chart outlines the average BMR for both men and women to give a general guideline for the number of calories you need to consume in order to lose weight. If you are at a healthy weight, do not cut your calories, but if you need to drop weight, reduce the applicable number in the chart by 500 calories per day. For example, if you have a medium activity level and weigh 200 pounds, you should eat 1,530 calories per day. The principle of weight loss is to take in fewer calories than you expend. This strategy will promote a healthy one- to two-pound loss per week.

Calculating Your Body Mass Index (BMI)

| | WEIGHT | | | | | | | | | | | | | | | |
HEIGHT	100	110	120	130	140	150	160	170	180	190	200	210	220	230	240	250
5'0"	20	21	23	25	27	29	31	33	35	37	39	41	43	45	47	49
5'1"	19	21	23	25	26	28	30	32	34	36	38	40	42	43	45	47
5'2"	18	20	22	24	26	27	29	31	33	35	37	38	40	42	44	46
5'3"	18	19	21	23	25	27	28	30	32	34	35	37	39	41	43	44
5'4"	17	19	21	22	24	26	27	29	31	33	34	36	38	39	41	43
5'5"	17	18	20	22	23	25	27	28	30	32	33	35	37	38	40	42
5'6"	16	18	19	21	23	24	26	27	29	31	32	34	36	37	39	40
5'7"	16	17	19	20	22	23	25	27	28	30	31	33	34	36	38	39
5'8"	15	17	18	20	21	23	24	26	27	29	30	32	33	35	36	38
5'9"	15	16	18	19	21	22	24	25	27	28	30	31	32	34	35	37
5'10"	14	16	17	19	20	22	23	24	26	27	29	30	32	33	34	36
5'11"	14	15	17	18	20	21	22	24	25	26	27	28	30	32	33	35
6'0"	14	15	16	18	19	20	22	23	24	26	27	28	30	31	33	34
6'1"	13	15	16	17	18	20	21	22	24	25	26	28	29	30	32	33
6'2"	13	14	15	17	18	19	21	22	23	24	26	27	28	30	31	32
6'3"	12	14	15	16	17	19	20	21	22	24	25	26	27	29	30	31
6'4"	12	13	15	16	17	18	19	21	22	23	24	26	27	28	29	30

Source: www.health.harvard.edu/topic/BMI-Calculator

Calculating Your Basal Metabolic Rate

WEIGHT	RESTING CALORIES	LOW ACTIVITY	MEDIUM ACTIVITY	HIGH ACTIVITY
100	1120	1450	1570	1680
110	1150	1490	1600	1720
120	1190	1550	1670	1780
130	1220	1580	1700	1830
140	1250	1630	1750	1880
150	1280	1660	1800	1920
160	1320	1720	1850	1980
170	1350	1750	1890	2000
180	1380	1790	1930	2070
190	1420	1850	1990	2100
200	1450	1880	2030	2180
210	1480	1950	2050	2200
220	1512	1970	2100	2270
230	1540	2000	2160	2300
240	1580	2050	2200	2400
250	1610	2090	2250	2410
260	1640	2130	2300	2460
270	1676	2170	2350	2500
280	1710	2220	2400	2560
290	1740	2260	2440	2600
300	1770	2480	2500	2660

EXERCISE RECOMMENDATIONS

Exercising does not have to be hard or intense to be beneficial. Moderately intense aerobic exercise raises your heart rate enough so that you break into a sweat. While exercising moderately, you should be able to carry on a conversation. (It is difficult to talk during vigorous aerobic exercise, which raises your heart rate significantly.)

The DASH diet recommends exercising a minimum of 30 minutes at least five times a week, but it's even better if you do moderate activity seven days a week for at least 30 minutes. You should build this activity level up as the weeks go by and try alternative exercises to build your whole body's fitness, such as weight training, cardiovascular exercises, and a component to improve your sense of balance. You should do cardiovascular or aerobic exercise every day when on the DASH diet. This activity could include:

* Walking (to work, to do errands, with your dogs or kids, up the stairs instead of using the elevator)
* Biking
* Swimming
* Sports
* Jogging
* Dancing
* Gardening
* Skiing
* Skating
* Organized sports (soccer, tennis, etc.)

Weight training should be incorporated into your exercise routine as soon as physically possible, this activity tones and build your muscles and strengthens your bones. Muscles use far more calories at rest than fat, so as you increase your muscles, you will burn more fat, which supports weight-loss goals. Exercise such as yoga is a great activity because it improves your balance and flexibility while reducing stress.

Many people think they have no time for exercise, but it is a matter of making it a priority. Pick a time that is unlikely to be cancelled when other commitments and responsibilities take precedence, like early in the morning. The key to success with exercise is to find an activity or an array of activities you can do almost any day, every day, for the rest of your life. And choose things you think are fun, because if it is not fun, you are less likely to stick with it.

Many people have discovered that they stick to an exercise program with enthusiasm if they keep a weekly exercise log. Keeping this record can also help you relate your exercising habits with your weight-loss results.

EXERCISE LOG

WEEK:

DAY OF THE WEEK	EXERCISE	DURATION / WEIGHT
Monday		
Tuesday		
Wednesday		
Thursday		
Friday		
Saturday		
Sunday		

Understanding Your Blood Pressure

SYSTOLIC (top number) in mm Hg		DIASTOLIC (bottom number) in mm Hg	CLASSIFICATION
50–90	combined with	35–60	Hypotension (low blood pressure)
90–100	combined with	60–65	Low normal
100–130	combined with	65–85	Normal
130–140	combined with	85–90	High normal
140–160	combined with	90–100	Hypertension (high blood pressure) mild stage 1
160–180	combined with	100–110	Hypertension (high blood pressure) moderate stage 2
180–210	combined with	110–120	Hypertension (high blood pressure) severe stage 3
210–240	combined with	120–140	Hypertension (high blood pressure) very severe stage 4

WHAT IT MEANS AND WHAT TO DO

You might feel tired, dizzy, weak, and even faint. You should increase your fluid intake and increase your potassium and salt intake.

Athletes and children often fall within this range. Simply adopt a healthy lifestyle to maintain this level.

The optimum blood pressure is thought to be 120/80. Maintain a healthy lifestyle, which includes regular exercise and the DASH diet

Adopt a healthy eating plan such as DASH to reduce blood pressure into a lower normal range.

This is not a range that usually requires medication, but adopting a healthy eating plan such as DASH and exercising will reduce this level to the normal range. Consult your doctor for the best strategy.

Can lead to strokes, heart attacks, heart failure, or kidney disease. Medication and adopting a healthy lifestyle is the best strategy to reduce blood pressure to a normal range. High blood pressure can have no symptoms, so it is important to get it monitored by your doctor.

Can lead to strokes, heart attacks, heart failure, or kidney disease. Medication and adopting a healthy lifestyle is the best strategy to reduce blood pressure to a normal range. Make lifestyle changes to help reduce your blood pressure, such as stop smoking, avoid stress, and limit alcohol consumption. High blood pressure can have no symptoms, so it is important to get it monitored by your doctor.

Can lead to strokes, heart attacks, heart failure, or kidney disease. Medication and adopting a healthy lifestyle is the best strategy to reduce blood pressure to a normal range. Make lifestyle changes to help reduce your blood pressure, such as stop smoking, avoid stress, and limit alcohol consumption. Symptoms of very severe blood pressure can include headache, chest pain, vision disturbances, irregular heartbeat, and blood in the urine.

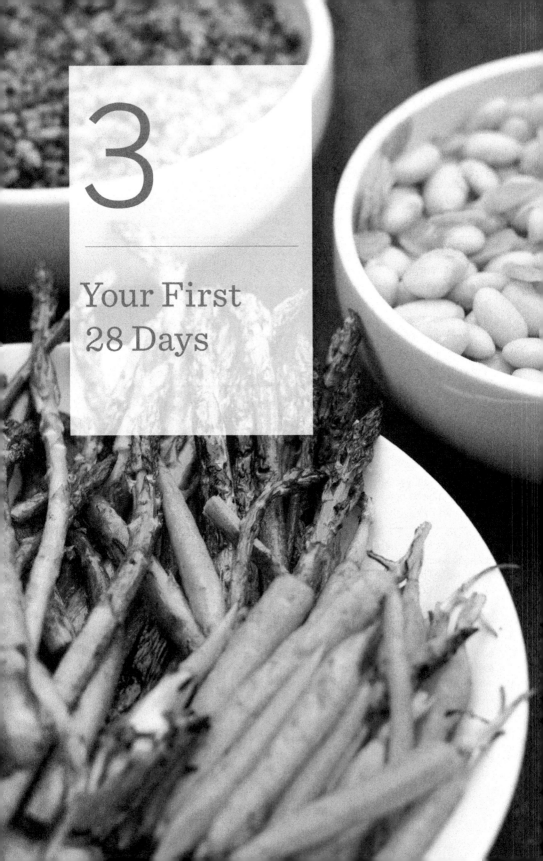

3

Your First
28 Days

TAKE THE TIME TO PLAN MEALS

Taking a few minutes to develop a meal plan for each day and each week is important for your DASH success. Once you put meal planning into your schedule, it becomes routine and makes it more likely that you will continue DASH, continue healthful eating, and continue on the path to health and wellness.

Planning ahead reduces the stress of meal planning and provides you with the proper tools to put a healthy meal on the table three times each day. If you know what you will cook on Monday, you can plan to eat leftovers on Tuesday and not cook again until Wednesday. Perhaps during the time you don't spend cooking, you can go for a walk.

Aunt Viv's birthday party on Saturday? No problem! Plan your meals with slightly fewer calories in the days beforehand so you can enjoy a small slice of birthday cake. Soccer game with the kids on Sunday? Your advance planning means you can pack a bag with healthful snacks and drinks for everyone.

Many of the recipes in this book are designed for four portions. Plan for leftovers to save time and effort. Just be sure to include the leftovers in your meal plan. Once you get into a routine that works for you and your family, keep at it. And remember, no one is perfect. There will be some days or weeks when even the best-laid plans go awry. When that happens, ask for help if you need it to get back on track.

STOCKING YOUR DASH DIET KITCHEN

Setting up your pantry to live the DASH lifestyle is very straightforward. It does not mean eliminating all sodium and fat from your diet, but it does mean reducing the overall amount of sodium and fat to improve your health. You can reduce sodium in packaged foods as well as table salt, and you can reduce the fats found in nuts, oils, dairy, and meat.

A balanced low-fat diet involves eating proteins, fats, and carbohydrates. Most people who follow the DASH diet do not have any problem getting enough of these nutrients in their daily routine, but if you have specific dietary needs, check with your doctor before switching to a DASH diet.

Each ingredient in your pantry should be nutrient-dense. Whole fats can include healthful oils such as olive and flax oil, fatty fish such as wild salmon and mackerel, and foods with reduced fat such as low-fat dairy, or egg whites instead of egg yolks.

Some cuts of meat are lower in fat than others. Chicken skin is notoriously fatty and does not belong in your low-fat pantry, but white meat is welcome. Slower-cooking cuts of meat, such as stew meat and ribs, are often marbled with fat. Ask your butcher to trim these down for you, or select a quicker-cooking, less fatty part of the animal. A knowledgeable butcher can give you options.

We all need some fat for optimum health, but by reducing fats and keeping lower-fat options nearby, we can easily reduce our overall intake. The following are many of the foods you'll need to make the recipes in this book. Having them on hand will make it easy to prepare your favorite meals.

FOR THE PANTRY

Jars, Boxes & Cans

Rice milk	Low-fat evaporated milk
Almond milk	Dried fruits—cherries, golden
Coconut milk	raisins, apricots, currants, figs

Almond butter

Peanut butter

Roasted hazelnut-chocolate
   spread

Canned pineapple chunks

Canned pumpkin purée

Jarred minced ginger

Tahini

Artichoke hearts packed
   in water

Low-salt vegetable broth

Low-salt, low-fat beef broth

Low-salt tomato purée
   or sauce

Low-salt diced tomatoes

Dijon mustard

Low-salt tamari or soy sauce

Sambal oelek or garlic
   chili sauce

Water chestnuts

Hoisin sauce

Barbecue sauce

Produce

Garlic

Yellow onions

Shallots

Sweet potatoes

Waxy potatoes such as
   Yukon Gold

Butternut and acorn squash

Fresh ginger

Grains & Legumes

Brown rice or wild rice blend

Whole-grain buckwheat

Whole-grain pasta

Corn tortillas

Quinoa

Rolled oats

All-purpose flour

Whole wheat flour

Cornmeal

Grits

Whole grain pita chips

Canned low- or
   no-salt chickpeas

Canned low- or no-salt
   cannellini beans

Canned low- or no-salt
   refried beans

Canned low- or no-salt
   black beans

Canned low- or no-salt
black-eyed peas
Canned low- or no-salt
pinto beans
Lentils
Quick-cooking and rolled oats
Popcorn
Pine nuts

Walnuts
Pecans
Sunflower seeds
Cashews
Pistachios
Flaxseeds
Sesame seeds
Pumpkin seeds

Oil and Vinegar

Extra-virgin olive oil
Flaxseed oil (needs to be
refrigerated once opened)
Canola oil
Grape seed oil
Coconut oil
Sesame oil

Walnut oil
White vinegar
Balsamic vinegar
Apple cider vinegar
Unseasoned rice vinegar
Red wine vinegar

Sweeteners & Flavorings

Maple syrup
Vanilla extract
Honey
70% cocoa dark chocolate

Unsweetened cocoa powder
Granulated stevia
Blackstrap molasses

FOR THE REFRIGERATOR

In addition to the preceding meat, fish, and dairy products, keep your fridge stocked with fresh vegetables and fruits. They are important sources of micronutrients, and they're loaded with fiber to help you feel full. Fresh herbs can add a lot of flavor at little cost.

These days there are low-fat versions of just about everything, even butter. Experiment with lower-fat versions of your favorite foods to find the ones you like best.

Dairy

Low-fat plain or plain
 Greek yogurt
Low-fat or skim milk
Low-fat cheese—blue, cheddar,
 Feta, ricotta
Part-skim mozzarella
Low-salt Parmesan

Goat cheese
Low-fat Swiss
Neufchatel or low-fat
 cream cheese
Low-fat sour cream
Egg whites

Produce

Fresh fruits—blueberries, bananas, limes, lemons, apples, melon,
 pears, grapes, strawberries, peaches
Fresh vegetables—kale, green onions, leeks, tomatoes, avocado,
 spinach, broccoli, cabbage, celery, green beans, carrots, zucchini,
 cauliflower, Japanese eggplant, bell peppers, asparagus, tomato,
 jicama, cucumber, fennel, endive, romaine lettuce, Bibb lettuce
Fresh herbs—cilantro, parsley, tarragon, basil, thyme, mint
Fresh chilis—jalapeño, pasilla
Orange juice
Silken tofu
Spelt bread

FOR THE FREEZER

Most people underuse their freezer, but it can help add value and variety to your cooking routine. You can purchase fruits and vegetables in season, when they are least expensive, and freeze them for later use. You can freeze leftovers in portion sizes and enjoy them later as a grab-n-go lunch.

Meat & Fish

Turkey bacon or vegan bacon

Skinless chicken breast

Chicken sausage

Ground turkey

Pork loin or lean ground pork

Buffalo

Lamb leg

Smoked salmon

Halibut

US-sourced shrimp

US-sourced yellowfin tuna

Canned, low-salt tuna packed
in water

Anchovies

Produce

Fruits—berries,
peaches, mangoes

Spinach

Broccoli

Corn

Peas

Green beans

Orange juice concentrate

Sliced spelt or millet bread

FOR THE SPICE RACK

Variety is the spice of life. Just a few spices, purchased in small amounts to ensure freshness, can make a huge difference in the flavor of your food. Purchase whole, unprocessed spices, and grind them yourself just before you cook, to ensure maximum flavor. Read the packaging labels to be sure you are purchasing powdered versions of spices and not spices with added salt.

Black peppercorns

Sea salt

Bay leaves

Cinnamon

Nutmeg

Ginger

Mace

White and black pepper

Sage

Marjoram

Oregano

Chili powder

Red pepper flakes

Cayenne

Garlic powder

Onion powder

Sweet paprika

Sweet smoked paprika

Dill

Cumin

Thyme

Curry powder

Turmeric

Coriander

Whole chile de àrbol

Poultry seasoning

Celery seed

Savory

Arrowroot powder

28-Day Meal Plan

This meal plan is specially designed to help you lose weight, so the total calorie count for each day is quite low. Feel free to add one additional snack and one dessert from the recipe section each day if you want more energy.

WEEK ONE

Congratulations on starting the DASH diet! Week one is usually the most challenging when committing to a new lifestyle because you are still entrenched in old habits. The fabulous news for you is that the DASH diet is not like other plans, so you will not have to stop eating entire food groups and spend hours preparing, weighing, and counting your food. DASH is all about delicious natural foods that will probably be familiar.

If you are a dedicated junk-food enthusiast or eat all your food from takeout windows, you might experience some side effects, such as cravings and headaches, during this first week. Don't despair, because these effects result from habits as well and will fade by the end of the week. The best strategy is to eat all the food and calories recommended on the DASH plan and incorporate exercise into the week at least five times. If you feel overwhelmed by cooking every meal instead of relying on convenience food, simply go for a walk, play with your kids, or turn the music on in your kitchen and dance. Celebrate your new lifestyle, and remember that food is supposed to bring you joy as well as nourish your body.

Monday

Breakfast: Store-bought fortified breakfast cereal with
fresh fruit and skim milk
Lunch: Waldorf Salad with Chicken
Dinner: Creamy Cheddar Grits with Shrimp
Snack: Hot Chocolate

Tuesday

Breakfast: Banana-Blueberry Smoothie
Lunch: Chicken Sausage and Quinoa Salad
Dinner: Tuna Salad Sandwiches
Snack: Hazelnut Spread and Banana Sandwich

Wednesday

Breakfast: Cream of Buckwheat Breakfast Cereal with
Fruit and Flaxseed
Lunch: Blue Cheese, Endive, and Apple Salad with
Walnut Vinaigrette
Dinner: Fish Tacos
Snack: Middle Eastern Hummus with Crudités

Thursday

Breakfast: Sausage and Egg Sandwich
Lunch: Cream of Tomato Soup with Fennel
Dinner: Grilled Skirt Steak with Salsa Verde
Snack: Kale Chips

Friday

Breakfast: Whole-Wheat Toast with Almond Butter and Apples
Lunch: Creamy Cauliflower Soup
Dinner: Lamb Kebabs with Garlic and Mint
Snack: Popcorn Without the Guilt

Saturday

Breakfast: Spring Vegetable Frittata
Lunch: Wild Rice Salad
Dinner: Buffalo Burgers
Snack: Dilly White Bean Dip

Sunday

Breakfast: Pumpkin Pancakes
Lunch: Cannellini Bean Salad with Mint and Parsley
Dinner: Pork Loin with Figgy Sauce
Snack: Artichoke-Feta Dip

WEEK TWO

Welcome to week two of your DASH diet journey. You should now be familiar with the DASH diet guidelines and be getting into a healthy eating routine. Keep in mind that slow, sustained weight loss, about two pounds per week, supports long-term success. If you have not dropped any weight yet, don't get discouraged. Eating nutrient-rich food low in calories and saturated fat will eventually produce the weight-loss results you desire.

You should feel more energetic and experience no sugar crashes in the afternoon because DASH recipes leave you satisfied, and their combined complex carbohydrates and protein digest slowly. You might find that you also sleep more soundly and wake up refreshed, because providing your body with abundant nutrients creates balanced hormones, including those that regulate sleep.

Your body should start losing the effects of eating a high-sodium diet, including bloating, puffiness in the face, and headaches. You might still crave old favorite indulgences such as chips or bacon, but your overall sense of well-being should diminish those feelings.

Monday

Breakfast: Sweet Potatoes and Pineapple
Lunch: Lentil Soup
Dinner: Bean and Vegetable Tacos
Snack: Spinach Dip with Basil and Water Chestnuts

Tuesday

Breakfast: Banana-Blueberry Smoothie
Lunch: Apricot Chutney and Cream Cheese on Toast
Dinner: Turkey Lettuce Cups
Snack: Peanut and Honey Protein Bar

Wednesday

Breakfast: Breakfast Tacos
Lunch: Minestrone with Pasta and Beans
Dinner: Tuna Salad Sandwiches
Snack: Artichoke-Feta Dip

Thursday

Breakfast: No-Cook Granola with Dried Fruit
Lunch: Onion Soup
Dinner: Chicken Dippers with Peanut Sauce
Snack: Pumpkin Dip

Friday

Breakfast: Whole-Wheat Toast with Almond Butter and Apples
Lunch: Chicken Noodle Soup
Dinner: Grilled Halibut with Spiced Yogurt
Snack: Traditional Baba Ghanoush

Saturday

Breakfast: Quiche with Asparagus, Salmon, and Tomato
Lunch: Leftover chicken and Coleslaw
Dinner: Black-Eyed Pea Burgers
Snack: Apricot Chutney and Cream Cheese on Toast

Sunday

Breakfast: Coconut Rice Pudding
Lunch: Chili with White Beans
Dinner: Turkey Sloppy Joes
Snack: Roasted Chickpeas

WEEK THREE

You are now no doubt becoming a DASH diet veteran, able to whip up smoothies and whole-grain cooked cereals in the morning while packing delicious lean meat wraps and fruit snacks for lunch. Healthy food choices should be exciting, but also start to be a habit in your daily routine. You will probably automatically order fresh salads with plain oil and vinegar dressing in restaurants while everyone else is consuming greasy French fries.

You should be adding extra exercise to your week as well, under a doctor's supervision, to speed your weight loss along. After this third week, there is a great chance that you have dropped at least five pounds and feel energized. Take this extra oomph and do a little spring cleaning or get a long-put-off task done in order to cleanse your environment and life along with your body.

You will find reading labels is now second nature, and you can pack your shopping cart with DASH diet choices more quickly than before. The organic section of the grocery store will contain fascinating ingredients you may never have tried before, such as quinoa, brown rice syrup, and exotic spices. Experiment with your taste profiles a bit, using products that meet the DASH guidelines and appeal to your palate.

Monday

Breakfast: Steel-cut oats with fresh fruit and skim milk
Lunch: Blue Cheese, Endive, and Apple Salad with Walnut Vinaigrette
Dinner: Broiled Curried Chicken and Yogurt Tenders
Snack: Kale Chips

Tuesday

Breakfast: Banana-Blueberry Smoothie
Lunch: Chickpea Wrap
Dinner: Ratatouille with Pasta
Snack: Dilly White Bean Dip

Wednesday

Breakfast: Whole-Wheat Toast with Almond Butter and Apples
Lunch: Minestrone with Pasta and Beans
Dinner: Fish Tacos
Snack: Plantains with Greek Yogurt and Honey

Thursday

Breakfast: Roasted Pears with Blue Cheese and Walnuts
Lunch: Waldorf Salad with Chicken
Dinner: Spicy Chinese Noodles
Snack: Hazelnut Spread and Banana Sandwich

Friday

Breakfast: Cream of Buckwheat Breakfast Cereal with
  Fruit and Flaxseed
Lunch: Potato Salad with Green Goddess Dressing and Herbs
Dinner: Speedy Turkey Chili
Snack: Traditional Baba Ghanoush

Saturday

Breakfast: Breakfast Tacos
Lunch: Open-Face Turkey and Pear Sandwich
Dinner: Pork Loin with Figgy Sauce
Snack: Corn chips

Sunday

Breakfast: Pumpkin Pancakes
Lunch: Wild Rice Salad
Dinner: Turkey Sloppy Joes
Snack: Guacamole

WEEK FOUR

You are now starting the last week of your first month on the DASH diet, so give yourself a pat on the back for the achievement! You might have slipped a few times during the month, but that is fine as long as you kept your goals in mind and got back on the plan. This is a lifestyle change, not a short-term fad diet, so be a bit flexible so you can stick to it.

You will feel a huge difference in your body by the fourth week on the DASH diet, and you should also see positive changes in your blood pressure and on the scale. Your healthy weight loss will be between five and eight pounds, depending on your activity level and calorie consumption. If your weight loss is slightly less than you want, try cutting down by about 200 calories per day and increasing your exercise intensity.

This week could be a wonderful time to start visiting farmers' markets and organic co-ops to find fresh produce choices and inspiration. After the fourth week, you might want to branch out with other recipes, so getting ideas from markets, online, and in this cookbook can help you expand your culinary repertoire.

Monday
Breakfast: Coconut Rice Pudding
Lunch: Chicken Noodle Soup
Dinner: Lamb Kebabs with Garlic and Mint
Snack: Popcorn Without the Guilt

Tuesday
Breakfast: Spring Vegetable Frittata
Lunch: Roasted Vegetable Wrap
Dinner: Wild Rice and Chicken–Stuffed Tomatoes
Snack: Apricot Chutney and Cream Cheese on Toast

Wednesday
Breakfast: No-Cook Granola with Dried Fruit
Lunch: Coleslaw
Dinner: Pork Tenderloin with Herbes de Provence
Snack: Roasted Chickpeas

Thursday

Breakfast: Quiche with Asparagus, Salmon, and Tomato
Lunch: Toasted Chicken and Apple Sandwich
Dinner: Vegetarian Kebabs
Snack: Hot Chocolate

Friday

Breakfast: Melon Salad with Ham and Berries
Lunch: Chicken Sausage and Quinoa Salad
Dinner: Buffalo Burgers
Snack: Middle Eastern Hummus with Crudités

Saturday

Breakfast: Sausage and Egg Sandwich
Lunch: Cream of Tomato Soup with Fennel
Dinner: Grilled Skirt Steak with Salsa Verde
Snack: Artichoke and Feta Dip

Sunday

Breakfast: Sweet Potatoes and Pineapple
Lunch: Fresh Salmon Salad Pita Pocket
Dinner: Creamy Cheddar Grits with Shrimp
Snack: Peanut and Honey Protein Bar

Set reasonable goals that are specific, measurable, and achievable. For example: "I want to lower my blood pressure to 120/80 and my LDL cholesterol to 129 milligrams." Or "I want to lose 10 pounds in the next six months."

Reward yourself for sticking with DASH, for losing that one pound a week, for exercising three times this week. Small rewards, like going to a movie or buying yourself a little present, are great for small achievements. If you set long-term goals, you can aim for bigger rewards.

PART TWO

The Recipes

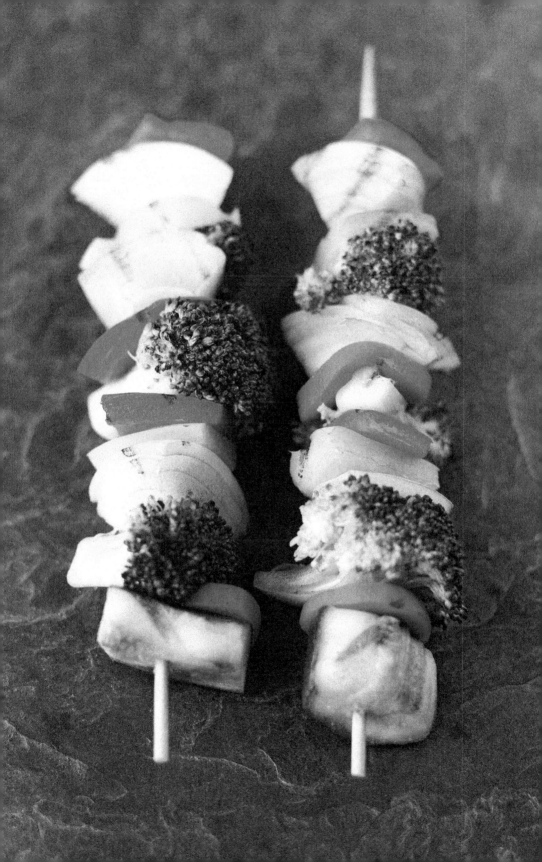

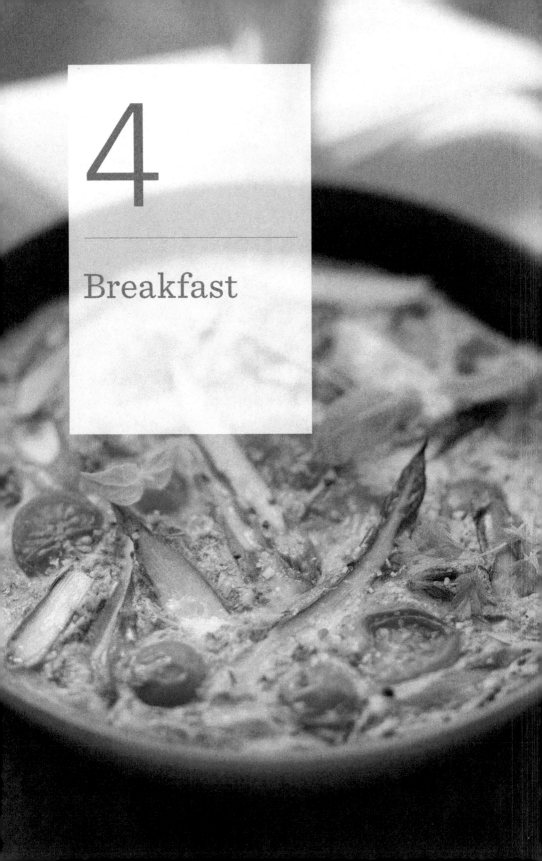

4

Breakfast

RECIPES

Banana-Blueberry Smoothie

This recipe is easily doubled or tripled. Experiment with other low-fat milks, such as soy or almond milk, until you find one with a texture and flavor you like.

1 cup frozen blueberries
1 banana
$\frac{1}{2}$ cup unsweetened low-fat cow's or rice milk
$\frac{1}{2}$ cup silken tofu

1. Combine berries, banana, milk, and tofu in a blender.

2. Blend until smooth and serve immediately.

Serves 1 PREP TIME: 5 MINUTES
PER SERVING: CALORIES: 133 FAT: 4.6 GRAMS CHOLESTEROL: 0 MILLIGRAMS
SODIUM: 89 MILLIGRAMS CARBOHYDRATES: 18.8 GRAMS
FIBER: 2 GRAMS PROTEIN: 1.8 GRAMS

Cream of Buckwheat Breakfast Cereal with Fruit and Flaxseed

This hearty cereal warms your body and soul on a chilly morning. Look for almond or rice milk that is low fat and fortified with calcium but does not contain added sugar or sweetener. Flaxseed oil is a monounsaturated fat and has a rich, full taste.

$2\frac{1}{2}$ cups fortified, unsweetened low-fat almond or rice milk
$\frac{1}{2}$ cup whole-grain buckwheat
$\frac{1}{4}$ cup coarsely chopped apples
1 tablespoon golden raisins
$\frac{1}{2}$ teaspoon cinnamon
$\frac{1}{8}$ teaspoon nutmeg
1 tablespoon flaxseed oil

1. Over medium heat, bring the milk to a simmer. Add buckwheat.

2. Return to a gentle simmer, reduce heat to low, and cook, partially covered, for approximately 10 minutes, stirring frequently, or until the milk is completely absorbed. Remove from heat.

3. Stir in apples and raisins, then allow cereal to rest for 5 minutes.

4. Stir in cinnamon, nutmeg, and flaxseed oil. Adjust seasonings as needed and serve.

Serves 4 PREP TIME: 15 MINUTES / COOKING TIME: 15 MINUTES
PER SERVING: CALORIES: 133 FAT: 4.6 GRAMS CHOLESTEROL: 0 MILLIGRAMS
SODIUM: 89 MILLIGRAMS CARBOHYDRATES: 18.8 GRAMS
FIBER: 2 GRAMS PROTEIN: 1.8 GRAMS

Coconut Rice Pudding

Make extra rice the night before and this dish comes together in minutes.

1 tablespoon orange-infused olive oil or plain olive oil
1 cup cooked long-grain rice
1 cinnamon stick
1 teaspoon vanilla extract
1 cup low-fat coconut milk
$\frac{1}{2}$ cup low-fat milk
$\frac{1}{2}$ cup dried cherries
$\frac{1}{2}$ cup toasted pecans
Pinch of ground nutmeg

1. In a medium sauté pan, heat oil over medium heat until warmed. Add cooked rice, cinnamon stick, vanilla, and coconut milk and stir to combine.

2. Bring to a simmer; then cook, partially covered over low heat, until coconut milk is absorbed, about 20 minutes. Remove from heat.

3. Add milk, cherries, almonds, and a pinch of nutmeg. Let rest, covered, for 10 minutes before serving. Add more milk if needed to achieve desired consistency.

Serves 4   PREP TIME: 5 MINUTES / COOKING TIME: 20 MINUTES
PER SERVING: CALORIES: 295 FAT: 25 GRAMS CHOLESTEROL: 0 MILLIGRAMS
SODIUM: 4.4 MILLIGRAMS CARBOHYDRATES: 35 GRAMS
FIBER: 5.7 GRAMS PROTEIN: 6.8 GRAMS

No-Cook Granola with Dried Fruit

Apricots have more potassium than bananas and make a nice change of pace. Prepare this granola in a to-go container and it "cooks" on your way to work.

1 $\frac{1}{4}$ cups low-fat milk

2 tablespoons honey

1 teaspoon vanilla extract

1 $\frac{1}{4}$ cups quick-cooking oats

$\frac{1}{2}$ teaspoon ground cinnamon

1 cup coarsely chopped dried apricots

1 cup chopped mixed unsalted nuts or seeds, such as walnuts, cashews, pecans, or sunflower seeds

1. Stir together milk, honey, and vanilla extract until combined. Add oats, stir to combine, and let rest for 15 minutes.

2. Add cinnamon and apricots, and let rest an additional 5 minutes.

3. Add nuts and stir thoroughly to combine. Serve immediately.

Serves 4   PREP TIME: 5 MINUTES / COOKING TIME: 20 MINUTES
PER SERVING: CALORIES: 424 FAT: 22 GRAMS CHOLESTEROL: 1.3 MILLIGRAMS
SODIUM: 30 MILLIGRAMS CARBOHYDRATES: 53.2 GRAMS
FIBER: 6.9 GRAMS PROTEIN: 10.9 GRAMS

Whole-Wheat Toast with Almond Butter and Apples

This is the grown-up version of peanut butter and jelly. Since this recipe calls for fresh apples, you're getting plenty of flavor and much less sugar than you would from jelly or jam.

4 slices spelt bread
4 tablespoons almond butter
1 apple, cored and cut into ¼-inch slices

1. Toast bread.

2. Spread 1 tablespoon almond butter onto each slice of bread.

3. Top with apple slices and serve.

Serves 4   PREP TIME: 5 MINUTES / COOKING TIME: 3 MINUTES
PER SERVING: CALORIES: 193 FAT: 9.6 GRAMS CHOLESTEROL: 0 MILLIGRAMS
SODIUM: 1.8 MILLIGRAMS CARBOHYDRATES: 25.4 GRAMS
FIBER: 3.7 GRAMS PROTEIN: 5.5 GRAMS

Melon Salad with Ham and Berries

This dish is a riff on the classic Italian prosciutto and melon salad. A spritz of lemon juice aids the absorption of vitamins and minerals.

Cooking spray
4 slices prosciutto
1 honeydew melon or cantaloupe, rind removed,
    chopped into ½-inch chunks
1 cup blueberries
4 lemon wedges

1. Preheat oven to 400°F. Spray a baking sheet with cooking spray.

2. Place prosciutto in a single layer on baking sheet. Bake for 8 minutes, or until crisp. Remove from oven and cool. Crumble.

3. Divide melon among four bowls. Add ¼ cup berries and a lemon wedge to each bowl.

4. Sprinkle crumbled prosciutto over fruit. Serve.

Serves 4   PREP TIME: 5 MINUTES / COOKING TIME: 10 MINUTES
PER SERVING: CALORIES: 154 FAT: 1.7 GRAMS CHOLESTEROL: 5 MILLIGRAMS
SODIUM: 243.1 MILLIGRAMS CARBOHYDRATES: 34.7 GRAMS
FIBER: 3.6 GRAMS PROTEIN: 3.4 GRAMS

Roasted Pears with Blue Cheese and Walnuts

Roasting pears brings out their sweetness, and blue cheese and walnuts are a classic accompaniment.

4 Bosc or d'Anjou pears, cored and quartered, skin on
1 tablespoon canola or grape seed oil
1 tablespoon lemon juice
Cooking spray
1/4 cup crumbled low-fat blue cheese
1/4 cup coarsely chopped toasted walnuts

1. Preheat oven to 425°F.

2. In a medium bowl, toss pears with oil and lemon juice.

3. Spray baking sheet with cooking spray, and place pears, cut-side down, on sheet. Roast for 15 minutes. Turn pears cut-side up and roast 10 more minutes.

4. Remove from oven. Divide pears among four plates, and top each serving with 1 tablespoon cheese and 1 tablespoon nuts. Serve immediately.

Serves 4   PREP TIME: 5 MINUTES / COOKING TIME: 25 MINUTES
PER SERVING: CALORIES: 200 FAT: 11 GRAMS CHOLESTEROL: 5 MILLIGRAMS
SODIUM: 66 MILLIGRAMS CARBOHYDRATES: 26.5 GRAMS
FIBER: 0.5 GRAM PROTEIN: 4.4 GRAMS

Sweet Potatoes and Pineapple

Pineapple is a good source of potassium and B vitamins. It contains the enzyme bromelain, which is thought to have anti-inflammatory properties. It is a natural complement to sweet potatoes.

2 tablespoons coconut oil or olive oil
4 baked sweet potatoes, sliced in half lengthwise
1 cup pineapple chunks, drained

1. Heat oil over medium-high in a large nonstick pan. Add sweet potatoes, flesh-side down, to pan.

2. Cook until the potatoes begin to brown and caramelize, about 8 minutes.

3. Place sweet potatoes on plates and top with pineapple. Serve.

Serves 4   PREP TIME: 5 MINUTES / COOKING TIME: 10 MINUTES
PER SERVING: CALORIES: 233 FAT: 7.2 GRAMS CHOLESTEROL: 0 MILLIGRAMS
SODIUM: 17.5 MILLIGRAMS CARBOHYDRATES: 41.3 GRAMS
FIBER: 4.4 GRAMS PROTEIN: 2.4 GRAMS

Pumpkin Pancakes

Pumpkin is loaded with potassium. One serving (two pancakes) delivers over 600 milligrams, about one-fourth of the recommended daily allowance.

$\frac{1}{2}$ cup all-purpose flour

1 cup whole-wheat flour

$\frac{1}{2}$ cup quick-cooking oats or oat flour

2 teaspoons baking powder

1 teaspoon pumpkin pie spice

4 egg whites

1 cup plain low-fat yogurt

1 teaspoon vanilla extract

$\frac{3}{4}$ cup low-fat milk

1 cup canned pumpkin purée

Cooking spray or olive oil

Low-fat sour cream for serving

1 apple, cored and sliced into $\frac{1}{2}$-inch pieces

1. In a medium bowl, mix together the flours, oats, baking powder, and pumpkin pie spice.

2. In a large bowl, combine the egg whites, yogurt, vanilla extract, milk, and pumpkin purée. Using a spatula, slowly incorporate the dry ingredients into the wet ingredients.

3. Heat a nonstick griddle or frying pan over medium heat. Spray pan with cooking spray or brush with olive oil.

4. When griddle is hot, add ⅓ cup of the batter to pan. Cook 3 minutes, or until small bubbles appear on the surface of the pancake. Flip and cook for another minute. Continue until all the pancakes are cooked. Serve with sour cream and apples.

Serves 4   PREP TIME: 10 MINUTES / COOKING TIME: 10 MINUTES
PER SERVING: CALORIES: 300 FAT: 2.6 GRAMS CHOLESTEROL: 4.7 MILLIGRAMS
SODIUM: 147 MILLIGRAMS CARBOHYDRATES: 54 GRAMS
FIBER: 7 GRAMS PROTEIN: 17.5 GRAMS

Breakfast Tacos

Unless you're from Texas, you probably don't think of tacos as a breakfast food, but these egg white and turkey bacon tacos make a tasty, high-protein start to the day. Cooking the bacon the night before simplifies preparation.

1 tablespoon olive oil
8 egg whites
4 corn tortillas
4 slices low-fat turkey bacon, cooked
$\frac{1}{4}$ cup chopped tomato
1 avocado, sliced

1. Heat olive oil in a medium, nonstick skillet over medium-high heat. Add egg whites and cook until set, about 2 minutes.

2. Warm tortillas according to package directions. Place one tortilla on each of four plates.

3. Top tortillas with eggs, bacon, tomato, and avocado and serve.

Serves 4   PREP TIME: 5 MINUTES / COOKING TIME: 15 MINUTES
PER SERVING: CALORIES: 210 FAT: 13.5 GRAMS CHOLESTEROL: 15 MILLIGRAMS
SODIUM: 343.2 MILLIGRAMS CARBOHYDRATES: 8.3 GRAMS
FIBER: 3.5 GRAMS PROTEIN: 13.9 GRAMS

Spring Vegetable Frittata

Although asparagus is available all year, it is most nutritious when it is in season, in the early spring. In fall, substitute cubed, cooked butternut squash and cooked Brussels sprouts. Jarred or defrosted frozen vegetables work equally well.

4 egg whites
1 teaspoon skim milk
1 tablespoon olive oil
1 handful of baby spinach leaves
4 cooked asparagus spears, chopped
¼ red bell pepper, chopped
Freshly ground pepper
1 ounce crumbled goat cheese

1. Preheat the broiler. In a small bowl, beat the egg whites with the skim milk until just combined.

2. Heat a small, nonstick, ovenproof skillet over medium-high heat. Add the olive oil, followed by the eggs.

3. Spread the spinach on top of the egg mixture in an even layer, and top with the asparagus and red pepper. Reduce heat to medium, and season with freshly ground pepper to taste. Cook the eggs and vegetables for 3 minutes, or until the bottom half of the eggs is firm and the vegetables are tender. ➤

Spring Vegetable Frittata *continued*

4. Top with the crumbled goat cheese, and transfer skillet to the middle rack under the broiler. Cook another 3 minutes, or until the eggs are firm in the middle and the cheese has melted.

5. Slice into wedges and serve immediately.

Serves 2   PREP TIME: 5 MINUTES / COOKING TIME: 15 MINUTES
PER SERVING: CALORIES: 162.7 FAT: 9.9 GRAMS CHOLESTEROL: 6.8 MILLIGRAMS
SODIUM: 215.5 MILLIGRAMS CARBOHYDRATES: 4 GRAMS
FIBER: 1.1 GRAMS PROTEIN: 14.7 GRAMS

Quiche with Asparagus, Salmon, and Tomato

This crustless quiche is light but remarkably filling, an ideal treat after a morning workout. It also makes delicious leftovers and is tasty cold or at room temperature.

1 tablespoon canola oil
1 cup chopped onion
6 asparagus spears, chopped into $\frac{1}{2}$-inch pieces
8 egg whites
$\frac{1}{2}$ cup shredded low-fat Cheddar
$\frac{1}{2}$ cup shredded low-fat mozzarella
$\frac{1}{4}$ teaspoon ground white pepper
4 ounces smoked salmon, chopped
Cooking spray
$\frac{1}{2}$ cup halved cherry tomatoes

1. Preheat oven to 350°F.

2. In a medium sauté pan, heat oil over medium-high heat. Add onion and asparagus, and sauté until onion begins to caramelize, about 8 minutes.

3. In a large bowl mix egg whites, cheeses, and white pepper. Gently mix in salmon. ➤

Quiche with Asparagus, Salmon, and Tomato *continued*

4. Pour egg mixture into a nonstick pie pan or pie pan coated with cooking spray. Add tomatoes, placing them in a circle around the outer edge of the egg mixture.

5. Bake for 30 minutes, or until eggs are set at the center. Allow to rest 5 minutes before serving.

Serves 8   PREP TIME: 10 MINUTES / COOKING TIME: 30 MINUTES
PER SERVING: CALORIES: 10 FAT: 4 GRAMS CHOLESTEROL: 8.9 MILLIGRAMS
SODIUM: 436 MILLIGRAMS CARBOHYDRATES: 4.6 GRAMS
FIBER: 1.1 GRAMS PROTEIN: 4.1 GRAMS

Sausage and Egg Sandwich

Making your own sausage is simple and allows you to eliminate most of the sodium. The herbs and spices give it plenty of flavor without salt. Double the recipe and put some in the freezer for later.

1 pound lean ground pork
$\frac{1}{2}$ teaspoon ground white pepper
1 teaspoon rubbed sage
$\frac{1}{2}$ teaspoon dried marjoram
$\frac{1}{2}$ teaspoon ground ginger
$\frac{1}{8}$ teaspoon ground nutmeg
Cooking spray
4 egg whites
4 whole-grain English muffins, split and toasted
4 slices low-fat Cheddar cheese
4 slices tomato
4 slices avocado

1. Combine the pork, white pepper, sage, marjoram, ginger, and nutmeg in a large bowl and mix well. Form into four patties.

2. Heat a nonstick griddle over medium heat. Spray griddle with cooking spray. Add patties to pan, and cook until well-browned and cooked through, about 8 minutes per side. ➤

Sausage and Egg Sandwich *continued*

3. Meanwhile, spray a small, microwave-safe bowl with cooking spray. Add egg whites and microwave on high until cooked through (about 2 minutes). Cook an additional 30 seconds if needed.

4. Place the English muffins on a plate and layer the cheese, tomato, avocado, sausage patties, and egg onto the muffins. Serve.

———————————

Serves 4   PREP TIME: 10 MINUTES / COOKING TIME: 20 MINUTES
PER SERVING: CALORIES: 375 FAT: 12 GRAMS CHOLESTEROL: 66 MILLIGRAMS
SODIUM: 532 MILLIGRAMS CARBOHYDRATES: 29 GRAMS
FIBER: 1.2 GRAMS PROTEIN: 40.3 GRAMS

Enlist the support of friends and family. Having people around you who can encourage you on tough days or cook a DASH meal for you when you cannot manage it yourself can be invaluable. It takes a village.

See the positive. Because DASH is designed for slow, steady, permanent weight loss, you may not see the changes you want as quickly as you anticipated. Celebrate your successes, no matter when or in what shape they arrive.

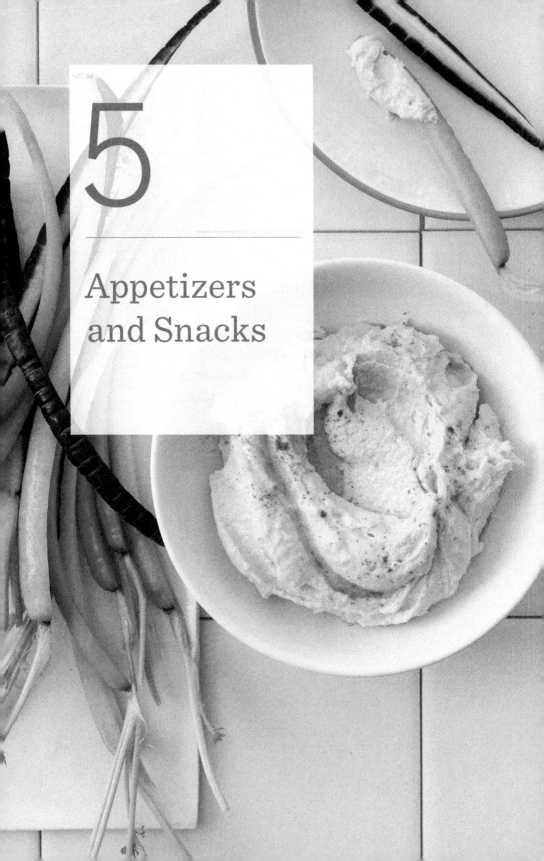

5

Appetizers
and Snacks

RECIPES

Hot Chocolate

Cocoa is rich in magnesium and antioxidants. A small amount of dark chocolate is heart-healthy and helps satisfy your craving for sweets. Look for chocolate that is about 70 percent cocoa. More than that and the chocolate will be quite bitter, and will not melt as easily.

4½ cups unsweetened low-fat almond milk
5 ounces dark or bittersweet chocolate (70 percent cocoa), chopped
¼ teaspoon ground cinnamon

1. Heat the milk in a saucepan over medium heat to just below the simmering point, reduce the heat to low, and add the chocolate. Stir gently to incorporate the chocolate into the milk.

2. When the chocolate is melted, add the cinnamon. Whisk vigorously and serve immediately.

Serves 4   PREP TIME: 5 MINUTES / COOKING TIME: 5 MINUTES
PER SERVING: CALORIES: 65 FAT: 4.3 GRAMS CHOLESTEROL: 0 MILLIGRAMS
SODIUM: 202 MILLIGRAMS CARBOHYDRATES: 4.4 GRAMS
FIBER: 0.3 GRAM PROTEIN: 1.4 GRAMS

Popcorn Without the Guilt

Popcorn at movie theaters and from microwave packages is often made with palm oil, an unhealthful saturated fat. Using an air popper at home seems retro, but it lets you control the added fat and seasonings. Make sure you use onion powder and garlic powder, not onion salt and garlic salt.

$1/2$ cup popcorn kernels
$1/2$ teaspoon onion powder
$1/2$ teaspoon sweet paprika
$1/4$ teaspoon garlic powder
$1/4$ teaspoon chili powder
2 teaspoons olive oil

1. Pop the popcorn using an air popper. While the machine is running, mix together the onion powder, paprika, garlic powder, and chili powder in a small bowl.

2. Place popped corn in a large bowl. Toss with olive oil, then with the spice mixture. Serve.

Serves 4   PREP TIME: 2 MINUTES / COOKING TIME: 5 MINUTES
PER SERVING: CALORIES: 50 FAT: 2.6 GRAMS CHOLESTEROL: 0 MILLIGRAMS
SODIUM: 0.3 MILLIGRAM CARBOHYDRATES: 6.2 GRAMS
FIBER: 1.2 GRAMS PROTEIN: 1 GRAM

Plantains with Greek Yogurt and Honey

For this dish, buy sweet yellow plantains, which often have brown blotches that indicate ripeness. You can find plantains in most grocery stores or at Latin markets.

2 tablespoon olive oil
2 yellow plantains, peeled and cut into 3/4-inch-thick slices
1/2 cup plain low-fat Greek-style yogurt, or other yogurt
1 tablespoon honey

1. In a medium nonstick sauté pan, heat olive oil until shimmering. Add plantains and cook until golden, about 5 minutes. Flip and cook for an additional 3 minutes. Remove from heat.

2. Combine yogurt and honey in a small bowl.

3. Drizzle plantains with yogurt mixture and serve.

Serves 4 PREP TIME: 2 MINUTES / COOKING TIME: 10 MINUTES
PER SERVING: CALORIES: 207 FAT: 8 GRAMS CHOLESTEROL: 1.3 MILLIGRAMS
SODIUM: 19.5 MILLIGRAMS CARBOHYDRATES: 32.9 GRAMS
FIBER: 1.8 GRAMS PROTEIN: 4.5 GRAMS

Apricot Chutney and Cream Cheese on Toast

This appetizer is incredibly portable—take it on your next picnic or have it on hand at work. For a satisfying lunch, add a slice of low-salt ham and a small salad.

$\frac{1}{2}$ cup chopped dried apricots

1 cup boiling water

$\frac{1}{4}$ cup currants

1 teaspoon jarred minced ginger

$\frac{1}{4}$ cup white balsamic vinegar

2 tablespoons granulated sugar

4 slices spelt bread

4 tablespoons low-fat cream cheese

1. Place apricots in a medium, nonstick sauté pan. Add boiling water and let sit 10 minutes. Add currants, ginger, vinegar, and sugar. Bring mixture to a simmer over medium-high heat.

2. Simmer for 20 minutes, stirring occasionally, until mixture begins to thicken. Remove from heat and cool.

3. Toast bread. Top with cream cheese and a thin layer of chutney. Serve.

Serves 4   PREP TIME: 10 MINUTES / COOKING TIME: 20 MINUTES
PER SERVING: CALORIES: 135 FAT: 3.2 GRAMS CHOLESTEROL: 8.4 MILLIGRAMS
SODIUM: 204 MILLIGRAMS CARBOHYDRATES: 24.1 GRAMS
FIBER: 1 GRAM PROTEIN: 4.9 GRAMS

Kale Chips

If you're looking for a crunchy snack to munch on instead of potato chips, you'll love these kale chips. If you are feeling lazy, roast the leaves whole. The stems are quite chewy.

2 heads curly leaf kale
2 tablespoons olive oil

1. Preheat oven to 325°F.

2. Tear the kale into bite-sized pieces, removing any tough stems, and place in a medium bowl. Add the olive oil.

3. Using your hands, massage the olive oil into the kale. When kale is glossy, lay it on a baking sheet in a single layer.

4. Bake for 10 to 15 minutes, or until crispy. Serve or store in an airtight container.

Serves 4   PREP TIME: 2 MINUTES / COOKING TIME: 10 MINUTES
PER SERVING: CALORIES: 70 FAT: 7.1 GRAMS CHOLESTEROL: 0 MILLIGRAMS
SODIUM: 8.8 MILLIGRAMS CARBOHYDRATES: 2 GRAMS
FIBER: 0.5 GRAM PROTEIN: 0.8 GRAM

Hazelnut Spread and Banana Sandwich

In many European countries, hazelnut-chocolate spread on toast is what's for breakfast. It is also a very portable snack. Bananas are a classic partner, but any seasonal fruit will do.

1 slice spelt or millet bread
1 tablespoon sugar-free hazelnut-chocolate or
    roasted hazelnut spread
2 tablespoons sliced banana

1. Cover bread with hazelnut spread.

2. Top with banana slices. Serve.

Serves 1   PREP TIME: 2 MINUTES
PER SERVING: CALORIES: 321 FAT: 6.6 GRAMS CHOLESTEROL: 0 MILLIGRAMS
SODIUM: 195.8 MILLIGRAMS CARBOHYDRATES: 62 GRAMS
FIBER: 6.5 GRAMS PROTEIN: 5.5 GRAMS

Middle Eastern Hummus with Crudités

Made from sesame seeds, tahini is often paired with chickpeas in Middle Eastern cuisine. Sesame seeds are loaded with calcium and magnesium as well as healthful fats. Try using this dip in place of mayonnaise on sandwiches.

Hummus

Two 15-ounce cans low-salt chickpeas, drained, rinsed, and slightly warmed

$\frac{1}{4}$ cup olive oil

Juice of 2 lemons

2 to 3 garlic cloves, coarsely chopped

$\frac{3}{4}$ cup tahini

$\frac{1}{4}$ teaspoon freshly ground pepper

$\frac{1}{2}$ cup toasted pine nuts (optional)

$\frac{1}{4}$ cup chopped flat-leaf parsley

Crudités

12 baby carrots

12 cherry tomatoes

12 jicama sticks

12 celery sticks, halved crosswise

1. Combine the chickpeas, olive oil, lemon juice, and garlic in a food processor and purée until smooth.

2. Add the tahini and pepper and continue to blend until creamy. If too thick, add a bit of water to thin it out. Place hummus in a serving bowl. Top with pine nuts and garnish with chopped parsley.

3. Serve with the crudités.

Serves 6   PREP TIME: 20 MINUTES
PER SERVING: CALORIES: 380 FAT: 26.4 GRAMS CHOLESTEROL: 0 MILLIGRAMS
SODIUM: 72.5 MILLIGRAMS CARBOHYDRATES: 29.6 GRAMS
FIBER: 9 GRAMS PROTEIN: 11.1 GRAMS

Guacamole with No-Salt Corn Chips

These classic chips and dip are made DASH-friendly by leaving out the salt. Avocados are loaded with healthy fats, and the rest of the fresh veggies add flavor and texture as well as nutrients.

Tortilla Chips
Cooking spray
4 corn tortillas, cut into triangles

Guacamole
2 avocados, cut into $\frac{1}{2}$-inch cubes
1 tablespoon lemon or lime juice
$\frac{1}{4}$ cup chopped tomato
$\frac{1}{4}$ cup chopped onion
$\frac{1}{4}$ cup chopped cilantro
$\frac{1}{4}$ cup peeled, seeded, and chopped cucumber

1. To make the tortilla chips, preheat oven or toaster oven to 325°F. Spray a small baking sheet or toaster tray with cooking spray. Place tortilla pieces on the baking sheet. Spritz tortilla pieces with cooking spray; bake 2 minutes, or until crisp.

2. To make guacamole, combine avocado and citrus juice in a medium bowl. Mash to blend. Add tomato, onion, cilantro, and cucumber and stir well.

3. Serve guacamole with chips.

Serves 6   PREP TIME: 15 MINUTES / COOKING TIME: 2 MINUTES
PER SERVING: CALORIES: 96 FAT: 8 GRAMS CHOLESTEROL: 0 MILLIGRAMS
SODIUM: 8 MILLIGRAMS CARBOHYDRATES: 28 GRAMS
FIBER: 4 GRAMS PROTEIN: 2 GRAMS

Dilly White Bean Dip

This dip tastes even better the next day, once the flavors have had time to develop. Rinsing the beans removes even more of the salt.

One 15-ounce can low-salt cannellini beans, rinsed and drained
1$\frac{1}{2}$ tablespoons lemon juice
$\frac{1}{2}$ cup low-fat sour cream
1 cup plain low-fat yogurt
1 tablespoon dried dill
1 teaspoon cumin
15 celery sticks
15 baby carrots
15 whole-wheat crackers or pita wedges

1. In a blender or food processor, combine beans, lemon juice, sour cream, yogurt, dill, and cumin, and pulse for one minute, until beans are broken down and all ingredients incorporated. Scrape down the sides if necessary.

2. Serve with celery sticks, carrots, and crackers.

Serves 8   PREP TIME: 20 MINUTES
PER SERVING: CALORIES: 87 FAT: 3.1 GRAMS CHOLESTEROL: 6.9 MILLIGRAMS
SODIUM: 131.1 MILLIGRAMS CARBOHYDRATES: 11.7 GRAMS
FIBER: 1.9 GRAMS PROTEIN: 5.7 GRAMS

Roasted Chickpeas

Almost any combination of spices works in this recipe, but the healthy dose of earthy cumin flavors the peas so nicely, you will not miss the salt.

Two 15-ounce cans low-salt chickpeas, drained and rinsed
2 tablespoons olive oil
1 teaspoon cumin
1 teaspoon dried thyme

1. Preheat oven to 400°F.

2. In a medium bowl, combine chickpeas, olive oil, cumin, and thyme. Toss to combine.

3. Spread chickpeas in a single layer on a jelly roll pan. Roast for 15 minutes, stir, and roast 15 minutes more.

4. Chickpeas are done when crisp outside and creamy inside. (Taste them to make sure!) Serve immediately.

Serves 8   PREP TIME: 5 MINUTES / COOKING TIME: 20 MINUTES
PER SERVING: CALORIES: 165 FAT: 5.5 GRAMS CHOLESTEROL: 0 MILLIGRAMS
SODIUM: 6 MILLIGRAMS CARBOHYDRATES: 23 GRAMS
FIBER: 6 GRAMS PROTEIN: 7 GRAMS

Traditional Baba Ghanoush

Serve this roasted eggplant spread with thin slices of hearty bread. You can also boost your vegetable servings by serving this tangy treat on cucumber rounds.

2 pounds Japanese eggplants
1 tablespoon olive oil
2 to 4 garlic cloves, peeled and minced
$\frac{1}{4}$ cup tahini
2 tablespoons lemon juice

1. Preheat broiler. Place oven rack at least 6 inches from heat source.

2. Cut eggplants in half lengthwise, and place on a broiler pan or lined baking sheet. Brush eggplants with olive oil. Broil eggplants, rotating pan once during cooking, 15 to 20 minutes, or until nicely charred and soft. Set aside to cool.

3. When eggplants are cool, scrape the inner flesh from the skins and transfer to a food processor. Discard skins. Add garlic, tahini, and lemon juice to food processor. Pulse until smooth, about 1 minute total, scraping down the sides of the bowl if needed. Serve or refrigerate.

Serves 4   PREP TIME: 10 MINUTES / COOKING TIME: 20 MINUTES
PER SERVING: CALORIES: 123 FAT: 11.5 GRAMS CHOLESTEROL: 0 MILLIGRAMS
SODIUM: 19.1 MILLIGRAMS CARBOHYDRATES: 3.7 GRAMS
FIBER: 1.4 GRAMS PROTEIN: 2.7 GRAMS

Artichoke-Feta Dip

If you have leftover roasted red bell peppers, use a small one here in place of the sun-dried tomato.

One 15-ounce can artichoke hearts, drained and coarsely chopped
$\frac{1}{4}$ cup (1$\frac{1}{2}$ ounces) crumbled low-fat feta cheese
1 sun-dried tomato, minced
$\frac{1}{4}$ cup chopped onion
1 garlic clove, minced
2 tablespoons lemon juice
1 tablespoon dried tarragon
$\frac{1}{4}$ teaspoon white pepper

1. Combine all ingredients in the bowl of a food processor. Pulse until coarsely chopped.

2. Serve immediately, or chill for up to three days before serving.

Serves 4   PREP TIME: 10 MINUTES / COOKING TIME: 20 MINUTES
PER SERVING: CALORIES: 116 FAT: 5.9 GRAMS CHOLESTEROL: 0 MILLIGRAMS
SODIUM: 193.7 MILLIGRAMS CARBOHYDRATES: 9.8 GRAMS
FIBER: 2.8 GRAMS PROTEIN: 6.3 GRAMS

Spinach Dip with Basil and Water Chestnuts

Pre-made spinach dip is widely available at grocery stores, but is loaded with salt and fat. This salt-free, low-cal version whips up quickly and will satisfy your cravings.

¼ onion, coarsely chopped

1 cup low-fat cottage cheese or ricotta cheese

½ cup baby spinach

¼ cup fresh basil, stems removed, torn into small pieces

One 8-ounce can sliced water chestnuts, drained and minced

½ teaspoon dried oregano

½ teaspoon dried marjoram

¼ teaspoon red pepper flakes

1 tablespoon olive oil (optional)

1. In the bowl of a food processor, combine onion, cheese, spinach, and basil. Pulse 1 minute to combine. Transfer to a medium bowl.

2. Stir in water chestnuts, oregano, marjoram, and red pepper flakes. If mixture is too thick, stir in olive oil. Serve immediately or refrigerate.

Serves 4   PREP TIME: 10 MINUTES / COOKING TIME: 20 MINUTES
PER SERVING: CALORIES: 90 FAT: 4.2 GRAMS CHOLESTEROL: 10 MILLIGRAMS
SODIUM: 230.7 MILLIGRAMS CARBOHYDRATES: 7.5 GRAMS
FIBER: 0.8 GRAM PROTEIN: 7.0 GRAMS

Peanut and Honey Protein Bar

The whole oats and nuts in this bar make a satisfying snack that will help you feel full between meals.

Olive oil or cooking spray
1 cup old-fashioned rolled oats
¼ cup unsalted peanuts
¼ cup unsalted sunflower seeds
1 tablespoon flaxseeds, preferably golden
1 tablespoon sesame seeds
1 cup unsweetened whole-grain puffed cereal
⅓ cup dried cranberries
⅓ cup chopped dried apricots
⅓ cup chopped golden figs
¼ cup unsalted creamy peanut butter
2 tablespoons brown sugar
¼ cup honey
½ teaspoon vanilla extract

1. Preheat oven to 350°F. Coat an 8-by-8-inch square pan with olive oil or cooking spray.

2. Spread oats, peanuts, sunflower seeds, flaxseeds, and sesame seeds on a large, rimmed baking sheet. Bake until the oats are lightly toasted and the nuts are fragrant, shaking the pan halfway through, about 10 minutes. Transfer to a large bowl. Add cereal, cranberries, apricots, and figs; toss to combine.

3. In a small saucepan, combine peanut butter, sugar, honey, and vanilla extract. Cook over medium-low heat, stirring frequently, until the mixture bubbles lightly, 2 to 5 minutes.

4. Immediately pour the peanut butter mixture over the dry ingredients, and mix with a spoon or spatula until no dry patches remain. Transfer to the prepared pan. Lightly coat your hands with cooking spray, and press the mixture down firmly to make an even layer (wait until the mixture cools slightly if necessary).

5. Refrigerate until firm, about 30 minutes. Cut into eight bars.

Serves 8   PREP TIME: 15 MINUTES / COOKING TIME: 10 MINUTES
PER SERVING: CALORIES: 209 FAT: 14.2 GRAMS CHOLESTEROL: 0 MILLIGRAMS
SODIUM: 41.6 MILLIGRAMS CARBOHYDRATES: 38.5 GRAMS
FIBER: 5.2 GRAMS PROTEIN: 8.1 GRAMS

Pumpkin Dip

This colorful, nutritious dip also makes a delicious sandwich spread.

1 tablespoon olive oil
$\frac{1}{2}$ yellow onion, finely chopped
2 garlic cloves, minced
One 15-ounce can pumpkin purée or cooked winter squash
1 teaspoon smoked sweet paprika
$\frac{1}{2}$ teaspoon ground cumin
$\frac{1}{2}$ teaspoon ground ginger
$\frac{1}{2}$ teaspoon curry powder
1 tablespoon water (optional)
1 tablespoon lemon juice
Unsalted pita chips

1. In a sauté pan, heat oil over medium heat. Add onion and garlic, and sauté until softened, about 6 minutes. Add the pumpkin and cook until hot, about 5 minutes.

2. Add paprika, cumin, ginger, and curry, and cook until spices have infused, about 2 minutes. Add a tablespoon of water if needed to prevent scorching.

3. Remove from heat. Add lemon juice, stir, and serve with pita chips.

Serves 4 PREP TIME: 10 MINUTES / COOKING TIME: 10 MINUTES
PER SERVING: CALORIES: 90 FAT: 3.7 GRAMS CHOLESTEROL: 0 MILLIGRAMS
SODIUM: 8.7 MILLIGRAMS CARBOHYDRATES: 13.9 GRAMS
FIBER: 4.3 GRAMS PROTEIN: 2.0 GRAMS

Keep track of your progress. Start a daily journal.
Write down what you eat and how you feel after you
eat. Write down how much you exercised and how you
felt after you exercised. Keep track of your mood or
anything else that seems important. After thirty days,
look back at what you wrote. Do you see any changes?
Where do you see success?

———————————————————

Keep setting goals. Goals provide a direction
and a plan and can help you stay focused. Don't beat
yourself up if you are not a perfect DASHer. Take a
look at your journal and see where you can
make changes.

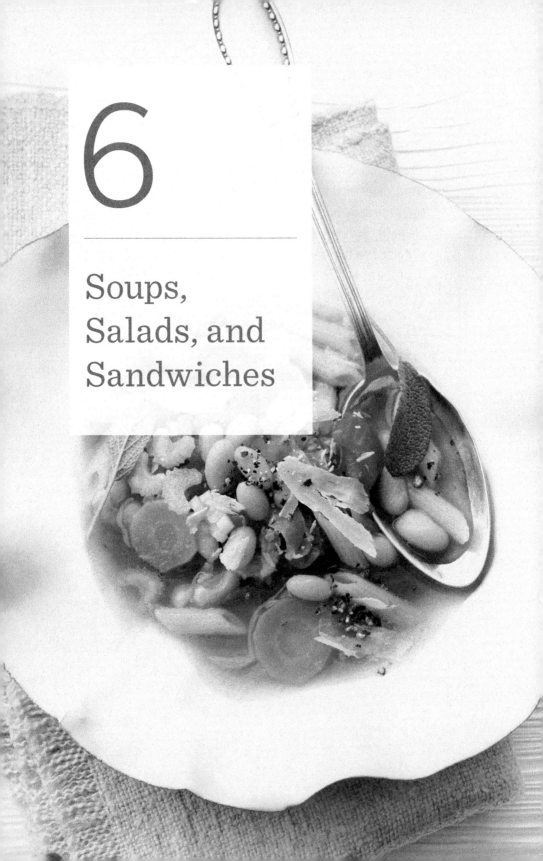

6

Soups, Salads, and Sandwiches

RECIPES

Creamy Cauliflower Soup

Evaporated skim milk boosts the calcium content of this soup and adds a nice creaminess without extra fat and calories.

2 tablespoons olive oil

1 cup chopped shallots (about 4 whole shallots)

4 cloves garlic, minced

2 teaspoons finely chopped fresh ginger

1 teaspoon curry powder

1 teaspoon ground turmeric

$\frac{1}{2}$ teaspoon ground cumin

$\frac{1}{2}$ teaspoon ground coriander

$\frac{1}{2}$ teaspoon freshly ground pepper

One 1-pound package pre-cut cauliflower florets

1 russet potato, peeled and cut into $\frac{1}{4}$-inch pieces

4 cups low-salt vegetable broth

1 cup evaporated skim milk

Chopped chives and low-fat sour cream for garnish

1. In a Dutch oven or large saucepan, heat oil over medium heat. Add shallots, garlic, and ginger and sauté, stirring frequently, until golden, about 5 minutes. Reduce heat to low and add curry, turmeric, cumin, coriander, and pepper. Stir 30 seconds, or until spices begin to release their fragrance.

2. Add cauliflower, stir to combine, and cook 2 minutes. Add potato and broth.

3. Increase heat to medium-high and bring soup to a boil. Cover and reduce heat to low. Simmer 20 minutes, or until cauliflower is tender.

4. Using an immersion blender, purée soup in the pot until smooth. (If you do not have an immersion blender, process in a traditional blender or food processor in batches, making sure to ventilate steam.) Whisk in milk.

5. Serve in bowls, topped with a teaspoon of chopped chives and a teaspoon of sour cream.

Serves 4   PREP TIME: 10 MINUTES / COOKING TIME: 20 MINUTES
PER SERVING: CALORIES: 204 FAT: 7.3 GRAMS CHOLESTEROL: 0 MILLIGRAMS
SODIUM: 223.9 MILLIGRAMS CARBOHYDRATES: 29.3 GRAMS
FIBER: 4.8 GRAMS PROTEIN: 8.2 GRAMS

Onion Soup

Onion soup is a classic French dish that is usually loaded with salt, and topped with toasted bread and fatty cheese. This DASH version eliminates the bread and cuts out much of the fat and sodium without sacrificing flavor, while adding chickpeas for protein.

1 tablespoon olive oil
2 sweet onions, sliced
2 cups chopped leeks, white and light green parts only
2 teaspoons granulated sugar
1 teaspoon chopped fresh thyme or ¼ teaspoon dried
4 cups low-salt, low-fat beef broth
One 15-ounce can low-salt chickpeas, drained and rinsed
¼ cup shredded low-fat Gruyère or Swiss cheese
Hot sauce for serving

1. In a large soup pot or Dutch oven, heat olive oil over medium-high heat. Add onions and leeks, and sprinkle with sugar. Reduce heat to medium and cook until onions and leeks are caramelized, 10 to 12 minutes.

2. Sprinkle onion mixture with thyme and cook, stirring, for 30 seconds. Add beef broth and chickpeas, and cook at medium-high heat until soup comes to a simmer, about 10 minutes.

3. Ladle soup into bowls. Top each bowl with 1 tablespoon cheese and serve with hot sauce.

Serves 4   PREP TIME: 5 MINUTES / COOKING TIME: 30 MINUTES
PER SERVING: CALORIES: 230 FAT: 6.9 GRAMS CHOLESTEROL: 7.8 MILLIGRAMS
SODIUM: 489 MILLIGRAMS CARBOHYDRATES: 33.4 GRAMS
FIBER: 5.3 GRAMS PROTEIN: 10.8 GRAMS

Cream of Tomato Soup with Fennel

Fennel, often used in Mediterranean cooking, is a natural digestive aid. It adds a delicate anise note to this soup.

3 tablespoons olive oil
1½ cups chopped yellow onions
1 fennel bulb, trimmed and chopped, fronds reserved
2 carrots, chopped
1 tablespoon minced garlic
One 28-ounce can low-salt tomato purée
1 tablespoon tomato paste
3 cups low-salt vegetable stock
2 teaspoons freshly ground pepper
¾ cup low-fat milk

1. Heat the olive oil over medium heat in a large, heavy-bottomed saucepan. Add the onions, fennel, and carrots and sauté, partially covered, until vegetables are quite tender, about 15 minutes. Add the garlic and cook for 1 minute.

2. Add the tomato purée, tomato paste, vegetable stock, and pepper and stir well. Bring the soup to a boil, lower the heat, and simmer, uncovered, about 15 minutes.

3. Whisk the milk into the soup. Serve garnished with reserved fennel fronds.

Serves 4   PREP TIME: 5 MINUTES / COOKING TIME: 30 MINUTES
PER SERVING: CALORIES: 260 FAT: 10.3 GRAMS CHOLESTEROL: 0.9 MILLIGRAM
SODIUM: 177.5 MILLIGRAMS CARBOHYDRATES: 34.6 GRAMS
FIBER: 2.6 GRAMS PROTEIN: 6.5 GRAMS

Minestrone with Pasta and Beans

In Italy, this soup is made with a Parmesan rind, which gives a pleasant richness to the stock but adds unnecessary sodium. Instead, sprinkle a bit of low-fat Parmesan on your soup at service.

1 tablespoon olive oil
1 chile de àrbol
1 cup chopped onion
1 cup diced carrot
1 cup diced celery
1 teaspoon dried oregano
$\frac{1}{2}$ teaspoon dried marjoram
$\frac{1}{2}$ teaspoon freshly ground pepper
1 cup low-salt cannellini beans, rinsed and drained
One 28-ounce can low-salt diced tomatoes with juice
1 cup low-salt vegetable stock
$\frac{1}{4}$ cup uncooked whole-grain pasta (small shapes, such as elbows or stars)
4 tablespoons grated low-fat Parmesan cheese

1. In a large sauté pan or Dutch oven, heat oil over medium-high heat. Add chile and cook 1 minute per side. Discard chile. Reduce heat to medium. Add onion, carrot, and celery and cook until onion is translucent, about 6 minutes.

2. Add oregano, marjoram, and pepper. Cook 30 seconds, until fragrant. Stir in beans, tomatoes with their juice, vegetable stock, and pasta. Turn heat to high and bring soup to a low boil; then reduce heat and cook 10 minutes, or until pasta is cooked.

3. Serve in bowls sprinkled with Parmesan.

Serves 4   PREP TIME: 5 MINUTES / COOKING TIME: 30 MINUTES
PER SERVING: CALORIES: 208 FAT: 4.6 GRAMS CHOLESTEROL: 5 MILLIGRAMS
SODIUM: 246.5 MILLIGRAMS CARBOHYDRATES: 33.6 GRAMS
FIBER: 4.8 GRAMS PROTEIN: 7.4 GRAMS

Chicken Noodle Soup

This classic soup is updated here with plenty of herbs. You can also add 1 cup chopped fennel or leeks for an extra serving of vegetables.

2 teaspoons olive oil
1 cup chopped celery
1 cup chopped carrot
$\frac{1}{2}$ cup chopped shallots
1 teaspoon salt-free poultry seasoning
4 fresh sage leaves, finely minced
$\frac{1}{2}$ teaspoon dried savory
$\frac{1}{2}$ teaspoon dried thyme
$\frac{1}{2}$ teaspoon celery seed
$\frac{1}{4}$ teaspoon white pepper
4 cups low-salt chicken broth
2 cups cooked chicken, cubed
1 cup cooked pasta
$\frac{1}{4}$ cup minced parsley

1. Heat oil over medium-high heat in a large saucepan or Dutch oven. Add celery, carrot, and shallots. Cook until shallots are translucent, about 6 minutes.

2. Add poultry seasoning, sage leaves, savory, thyme, celery seed, and white pepper, and cook 30 seconds.

3. Add chicken broth, turn heat to high, and bring to a low boil. Add chicken and pasta. Cook until warmed through, 5 minutes.

4. Ladle into bowls, sprinkle with parsley, and serve.

Serves 4   PREP TIME: 5 MINUTES / COOKING TIME: 30 MINUTES
PER SERVING: CALORIES: 180 FAT: 4 GRAMS CHOLESTEROL: 40.1 MILLIGRAMS
SODIUM: 167 MILLIGRAMS CARBOHYDRATES: 14.8 GRAMS
FIBER: 3 GRAMS PROTEIN: 16.6 GRAMS

Chili with White Beans

This recipe works beautifully with leftover roast chicken or turkey. Rinsing canned beans, even low-salt beans, removes even more sodium.

1 tablespoon canola oil

$1\frac{1}{2}$ cups chopped onion

Two 4-ounce cans low-salt chopped green chilies

1 teaspoon dried oregano

$\frac{1}{2}$ teaspoon dried marjoram

1 teaspoon ground cumin

$\frac{1}{8}$ to $\frac{1}{4}$ teaspoon cayenne pepper

Three 15-ounce cans low-salt great northern beans,
    rinsed and drained

4 cups low-salt chicken broth

4 cups diced cooked skinless turkey or chicken

2 tablespoons cider vinegar

$\frac{1}{4}$ cup grated low-salt Parmesan cheese

1. Heat oil in a large pot or Dutch oven over medium-high heat. Add onion and cook, stirring occasionally until softened, about 5 minutes.

2. Stir in chilies, oregano, marjoram, cumin, and cayenne. Cook, stirring occasionally, for 5 minutes. Stir in beans and broth; bring to a simmer. Cook, stirring occasionally, for 20 minutes.

3. Add turkey (or chicken) and vinegar; cook for 5 minutes more.

4. Ladle into four bowls. Sprinkle each bowl with 1 tablespoon of the Parmesan cheese. Serve.

Serves 4   PREP TIME: 5 MINUTES / COOKING TIME: 30 MINUTES
PER SERVING: CALORIES: 461 FAT: 8 GRAMS CHOLESTEROL: 55.2 MILLIGRAMS
SODIUM: 235 MILLIGRAMS CARBOHYDRATES: 53.8 GRAMS
FIBER: 16.6 GRAMS PROTEIN: 30 GRAMS

Lentil Soup

Jalapeño adds a warm spiciness to this dish. Leave it out, or substitute ¼ teaspoon cayenne pepper for less heat. Chopped leftover cabbage makes a nice addition.

2 teaspoons olive oil
1 cup chopped onion
1 cup chopped celery
1 jalapeño, seeded and finely chopped
2 cups chopped carrots
Two 15-ounce cans low-salt red or brown lentils, drained
4 cups water
One 15-ounce can low-salt tomato sauce
¼ teaspoon freshly ground pepper
¼ cup chopped fresh cilantro

1. Heat oil in a large soup pot over medium-high heat. Add onion, celery, jalapeño, and carrot. Cook until vegetables begin to soften, about 6 minutes.

2. Add lentils, water, tomato sauce, and pepper. Bring to a low boil; reduce heat and simmer 15 minutes, or until vegetables are tender.

3. Ladle into bowls and top with cilantro. Serve.

Serves 4   PREP TIME: 10 MINUTES / COOKING TIME: 20 MINUTES
PER SERVING: CALORIES: 150 FAT: 1 GRAM CHOLESTEROL: 0 MILLIGRAMS
SODIUM: 34 MILLIGRAMS CARBOHYDRATES: 28 GRAMS
FIBER: 25 GRAMS PROTEIN: 8 GRAMS

Chicken Sausage and Quinoa Salad

Quinoa contains an ideal mix of protein, carbohydrates, and fat to keep you full and energized for hours. Add whatever vegetables you have on hand and a quick dressing of oil and vinegar to make a quick meal.

2 cups water
1 cup quinoa
½ cup cooked sweet potato, cubed
2 scallions, minced
1 chicken sausage, cooked and cut into ½-inch slices
1 avocado, cut into ½-inch cubes
2 tablespoons sesame oil
1 tablespoon minced parsley

1. In a medium saucepan, bring 2 cups water to a boil. Add quinoa and cook, partially covered, over medium-low heat until most of the water is absorbed, about 20 minutes. Let quinoa rest for 5 minutes; afterwards spread it out on a jelly roll pan to cool.

2. Meanwhile, place the sweet potato, scallions, sausage, and avocado in a medium bowl. Toss with the sesame oil and parsley.

3. Add quinoa to the bowl and toss to combine. Serve.

Serves 4   PREP TIME: 10 MINUTES / COOKING TIME: 15 MINUTES
PER SERVING: CALORIES: 366 FAT: 18.5 GRAMS CHOLESTEROL: 15 MILLIGRAMS
SODIUM: 143 MILLIGRAMS CARBOHYDRATES: 41.5 GRAMS
FIBER: 7.4 GRAMS PROTEIN: 11.1 GRAMS

Blue Cheese, Endive, and Apple Salad with Walnut Vinaigrette

This sophisticated combination of flavors makes for a tasty and satisfying salad. It's colorful as well, and is a dish suitable for company.

$\frac{1}{4}$ cup red wine vinegar

3 tablespoons walnut oil

$\frac{1}{2}$ teaspoon Dijon mustard

1 tablespoon minced fresh tarragon

4 small heads white or red endive, cored and cut into 1-inch pieces

1 Yellow or Red Delicious apple, cored and cut into $\frac{1}{2}$-inch slices

4 cups romaine lettuce, torn into bite-size pieces

$\frac{1}{4}$ cup (1 ounce) crumbled low-fat blue cheese

1. In a small bowl, whisk together the vinegar, oil, mustard, and tarragon.

2. Place endive, apple, romaine, and blue cheese in a large salad bowl and toss gently to combine.

3. Divide salad equally among four plates. Drizzle each portion with 1 tablespoon of the dressing and serve.

Serves 4   PREP TIME: 15 MINUTES
PER SERVING: CALORIES: 240 FAT: 13.5 GRAMS CHOLESTEROL: 5.3 MILLIGRAMS
SODIUM: 310 MILLIGRAMS CARBOHYDRATES: 23.2 GRAMS
FIBER: 26 GRAMS PROTEIN: 9 GRAMS

Waldorf Salad with Chicken

The classic Waldorf salad features a mayonnaise-based dressing. Substituting nonfat yogurt for the mayo reduces salt and fat significantly. Using pistachios instead of the usual walnuts makes for an interesting change-up.

¼ cup plain nonfat yogurt
1 tablespoon olive oil
½ teaspoon curry powder
¼ teaspoon cayenne pepper
1½ cups 1-inch cubes of cooked chicken
1 cup halved seedless red grapes
1 cup chopped celery
⅓ cup golden raisins
⅓ cup unsalted pistachios, toasted and coarsely chopped
4 cups mixed baby salad greens

1. In a small bowl, whisk together the yogurt, olive oil, curry powder, and cayenne pepper.

2. In a large bowl, combine the chicken, grapes, celery, raisins, pistachios, and salad greens.

3. Divide salad evenly among four plates. Drizzle each portion with 1 tablespoon of the dressing and serve.

Serves 4   PREP TIME: 15 MINUTES
PER SERVING: CALORIES: 182 FAT: 6.6 GRAMS CHOLESTEROL: 19.1 MILLIGRAMS
SODIUM: 53.2 MILLIGRAMS CARBOHYDRATES: 22.9 GRAMS
FIBER: 2.3 GRAMS PROTEIN: 10.4 GRAMS

Carrot-Coconut Salad

Tamari is similar to soy sauce, but is typically lower in sodium and often gluten-free. A vegetable peeler with a julienne blade makes quick work of the carrots.

2 tablespoons honey

¼ cup orange juice

1 teaspoon minced ginger (fresh or jarred)

1 teaspoon low-salt tamari

1 tablespoon orange-infused oil or olive oil

2 cups carrots, grated or julienned

1 cup unsweetened coconut flakes

½ cup unsalted pecans or cashews, toasted and chopped

1. In a medium bowl, combine honey, orange juice, ginger, tamari, and oil.

2. Mix in carrots, coconut flakes, and nuts.

3. Toss until dressing evenly coats salad. Serve.

Serves 4 PREP TIME: 15 MINUTES

PER SERVING: CALORIES: 375 FAT: 25 GRAMS CHOLESTEROL: 0 MILLIGRAMS
SODIUM: 74.6 MILLIGRAMS CARBOHYDRATES: 32.7 GRAMS
FIBER: 3.2 GRAMS PROTEIN: 7 GRAMS

Coleslaw

This traditional-tasting salad contains no mayonnaise, and will quickly become a favorite. If pressed for time, you can use the prepackaged bags of sliced cabbage and carrot, but don't use packaged dressing.

⅓ cup white vinegar
3 tablespoons canola oil
1 tablespoon granulated sugar
1 teaspoon Dijon mustard
1 teaspoon celery seeds
4 cups thinly sliced cabbage
2 carrots, julienned
2 scallions, minced
2 celery ribs, minced

1. In a salad bowl, whisk the vinegar, oil, sugar, mustard, and celery seeds until well combined.

2. Add cabbage, carrots, scallions, and celery. Toss to combine.

3. Refrigerate 1 hour or up to 4 hours. Serve.

Serves 4   PREP TIME: 15 MINUTES
PER SERVING: CALORIES: 145 FAT: 10.8 GRAMS CHOLESTEROL: 0 MILLIGRAMS
SODIUM: 75.1 MILLIGRAMS CARBOHYDRATES: 12.2 GRAMS
FIBER: 3.8 GRAMS PROTEIN: 2.2 GRAMS

Wild Rice Salad

This salad is the essence of autumn. In the spring, substitute peas and asparagus for the squash and cranberries.

¼ cup walnut oil
¼ cup red wine vinegar
1 teaspoon Dijon mustard
1 small shallot, minced
2 cups cooked wild and brown rice blend
1 cup cubed cooked butternut squash
½ cup dried cranberries
½ cup pecans, toasted
4 cups mixed baby salad greens
1 cup baby spinach
¼ cup low-salt, low-fat Pecorino or mozzarella

1. In a small bowl, whisk together the oil, vinegar, and mustard. Add shallot and whisk to combine.

2. In a large salad bowl, combine rice, squash, cranberries, pecans, salad greens, spinach, and cheese. Toss to combine.

3. Divide salad evenly among four plates. Drizzle 1 tablespoon dressing on each portion. Serve.

Serves 4   PREP TIME: 15 MINUTES
PER SERVING: CALORIES: 344 FAT: 3.7 GRAMS CHOLESTEROL: 6.3 MILLIGRAMS
SODIUM: 195 MILLIGRAMS CARBOHYDRATES: 25.4 GRAMS
FIBER: 5 GRAMS PROTEIN: 5.3 GRAMS

Potato Salad with Green Goddess Dressing and Herbs

This salad plays up the fresh flavors of herbs. Adjust the ratios with the season, or substitute any other soft herbs. If avocados are out of season, vacuum-packed avocado or guacamole will do. If the buttermilk you have isn't tangy enough for your taste, add up to a tablespoon of white vinegar to it.

2 pounds waxy potatoes, peel left on, cut into 1-inch pieces
$\frac{1}{2}$ cup low-fat buttermilk
1 avocado
$\frac{1}{4}$ cup coarsely chopped fresh basil
$\frac{1}{4}$ cup minced fresh dill
$\frac{1}{4}$ cup minced fresh parsley
$\frac{1}{4}$ cup minced fresh mint
$\frac{1}{4}$ teaspoon white pepper
2 scallions, both white and green parts, minced
$\frac{1}{2}$ cucumber (about 1 cup), peeled, seeded, and chopped

1. Add potatoes to a large saucepan or Dutch oven, and cover with water by 1 inch. Bring to a boil over high heat; then turn off heat. Let potatoes rest for 5 minutes, and then drain and cool them. ➤

Potato Salad with Green Goddess Dressing
and Herbs *continued*

2. Meanwhile, add buttermilk, avocado, and basil to the bowl
of a food processor. Process for 2 minutes, or until smooth. Pour
dressing into a large salad bowl.

3. Add potatoes, dill, parsley, mint, pepper, scallions, and
cucumber. Toss to combine, and serve.

Serves 4 PREP TIME: 25 MINUTES / COOKING TIME: 5 MINUTES
PER SERVING: CALORIES: 189 FAT: 7.7 GRAMS CHOLESTEROL: 1.2 MILLIGRAMS
SODIUM: 41.5 MILLIGRAMS CARBOHYDRATES: 25 GRAMS
FIBER: 11.8 GRAMS PROTEIN: 6.3 GRAMS

Cannellini Bean Salad with Mint and Parsley

Any white bean works in this recipe. White beans have a neutral flavor, and take on the flavor of whatever you add to them. Artichokes, cherry tomatoes, and leftover cooked broccoli all make fine additions to the salad. Serve with Lamb Kebabs with Garlic and Mint (recipe on page 143).

¼ cup extra virgin olive oil
¼ cup minced fresh mint
¼ cup minced fresh parsley
1 anchovy, minced
1 garlic clove, minced
¼ cup minced red onion
Two 15-ounce cans low-salt cannellini beans or
    other white beans, drained and rinsed

1. In a medium bowl, combine olive oil, mint, and parsley. Add anchovy, garlic, and red onion.

2. Add beans to herb mixture and gently mix to combine. Serve.

Serves 4   PREP TIME: 10 MINUTES
PER SERVING: CALORIES: 246.8 FAT: 13.6 GRAMS CHOLESTEROL: 0.9 MILLIGRAM
SODIUM: 267.5 MILLIGRAMS CARBOHYDRATES: 26.6 GRAMS
FIBER: 8.2 GRAMS PROTEIN: 9.8 GRAMS

Open-Face Turkey and Pear Sandwich

This sandwich has a breezy bistro feel, especially if you enjoy it on a patio in the sun. It is important to use turkey breast that you roast yourself or find a product that is low in sodium, because prepared meats can contain a staggering amount of sodium. Serve this meal with a tossed green salad to keep the total sodium levels low.

4 slices low-sodium multigrain bread (or low-sodium rye)
4 teaspoons spicy Dijon-style mustard
2 ripe pears, cored and cut into thin slices lengthwise
4 ounces cooked turkey breast, cut thinly into 8 slices
2 ounces shredded low-sodium Swiss cheese
Freshly ground pepper

1. Preheat oven to broil.

2. Place bread slices on a baking sheet.

3. Spread 1 teaspoon of mustard evenly on each bread slice.

4. Divide pear slices among bread slices, layering so each slice is covered.

5. Top with two turkey slices each, and sprinkle with shredded cheese.

6. Place baking sheet on a rack about 4 inches from broiler heat, and broil sandwiches until cheese is melted and turkey is warmed, about 2 minutes.

7. Remove from oven and season with pepper. Serve hot.

Serves 4   PREP TIME: 10 MINUTES / COOKING TIME: 2 MINUTES
PER SERVING: CALORIES: 244 FAT: 8.4 GRAMS CHOLESTEROL: 25 MILLIGRAMS
SODIUM: 490 MILLIGRAMS CARBOHYDRATES: 32 GRAMS
FIBER: 6 GRAMS PROTEIN: 13 GRAMS

Roasted Vegetable Wrap

If you have a barbecue, you can grill your vegetables with wonderful results. Simply toss the cut-up vegetables with olive oil, and grill them until they are lightly charred and tender. Make sure you let your vegetables cool down at least 30 minutes, and shake off any excess liquid so that your wraps are not soggy.

2 tablespoons olive oil
1 teaspoon balsamic vinegar
1 small eggplant, cut into thin slices widthwise
1 medium green zucchini, sliced lengthwise
1 red bell pepper, seeded and cut into eight slices
1 small red onion, cut into $\frac{1}{4}$-inch slices
$\frac{1}{4}$ cup gently packed shredded basil
Two 8-inch whole-wheat tortillas
Freshly ground pepper

1. Preheat oven to 450°F. Line a baking sheet with foil.

2. Put olive oil, vinegar, eggplant, zucchini, bell pepper, and onion in a large bowl and toss until well combined. Transfer to baking sheet, and spread out evenly.

3. Place vegetables in oven, and roast until tender, turning once, about 20 minutes.

4. Remove from oven, and transfer to a bowl. Cool for 30 minutes.

5. Add shredded basil and toss to combine.

6. Lay tortillas on a clean work surface, and spread roasted vegetable mixture evenly, shaking off any extra liquid. Season with pepper.

7. Fold tortillas around roasted vegetables and serve.

Serves 2   PREP TIME: 10 MINUTES / COOKING TIME: 20 MINUTES
PER SERVING: CALORIES: 343 FAT: 15.8 GRAMS CHOLESTEROL: 0 MILLIGRAMS
SODIUM: 143 MILLIGRAMS CARBOHYDRATES: 46.6 GRAMS
FIBER: 14.9 GRAMS PROTEIN: 9.2 GRAMS

Fresh Salmon Salad Pita Pocket

This is a healthy twist on the classic mayonnaise-drenched tuna salad. It is high in heart-healthy omega-3 fatty acids and low in cholesterol. You can use canned salmon if you find a low-sodium product packed in water instead of oil, but fresh is best whenever possible. You can grill, bake, pan sear, or poach fresh salmon, depending on your preference.

8 ounces cooked fresh salmon
1 green onion, finely chopped
1 celery stalk, finely chopped
¼ red bell pepper, finely chopped
2 tablespoons plain fat-free yogurt
2 teaspoons lemon juice
1 teaspoon chopped fresh dill
Freshly ground pepper
½ cup gently packed shredded fresh spinach
2 small whole-wheat pita breads, cut in half

1. In a medium bowl, flake cooked salmon with a fork.

2. Mix in green onion, celery, bell pepper, yogurt, lemon juice, dill, and pepper. Combine well.

3. Fill four pita halves evenly with salmon salad and shredded spinach, and serve.

Serves 2   PREP TIME: 10 MINUTES
PER SERVING: CALORIES: 308 FAT: 8.9 GRAMS CHOLESTEROL: 51 MILLIGRAMS
SODIUM: 284 MILLIGRAMS CARBOHYDRATES: 30.4 GRAMS
FIBER: 5 GRAMS PROTEIN: 28.8 GRAMS

Toasted Chicken and Apple Sandwich

Cheddar cheese and apple is a tasty classic combination that works well with chicken breast and peppery arugula. This sandwich would also be fabulous grilled on the barbecue instead of toasted. Simply assemble the sandwich completely and brush the untoasted bread with a little olive oil before placing it on a medium-hot barbecue. Grill both sides and serve.

4 slices low-sodium multigrain bread
2 tablespoons low-fat mayonnaise
1 tart apple, cored and cut into thin slices
4 ounces cooked chicken breast, cut into 4 thin slices
2 slices low-sodium Cheddar cheese, about ¼ inch thick
1 cup gently packed shredded arugula

1. Toast bread until golden brown, and spread all four slices with mayonnaise.

2. Layer apple, chicken, and Cheddar cheese evenly on two slices of bread.

3. Top cheese with arugula and a second slice of toasted bread.

4. Cut sandwiches in half and serve.

Serves 2   PREP TIME: 10 MINUTES / COOKING TIME: 2 MINUTES
PER SERVING: CALORIES: 432 FAT: 17.6 GRAMS CHOLESTEROL: 80 MILLIGRAMS
SODIUM: 184 MILLIGRAMS CARBOHYDRATES: 40 GRAMS
FIBER: 4.4 GRAMS PROTEIN: 30.4 GRAMS

Chickpea Wrap

Chickpeas are loaded with protein and fiber. They make a fantastic sandwich filling and they are also perfect for achieving weight-loss goals, because research has shown that including these tasty legumes in your meals can reduce the consumption of processed foods and keep you satisfied longer.

One 16-ounce can low-salt chickpeas, drained and rinsed
1 stalk celery, finely chopped
¼ red onion, finely chopped
½ cup green grapes, halved
2 tablespoons plain fat-free yogurt
2 tablespoon chopped cashews
· 1 teaspoon curry powder
Two 8-inch whole-wheat tortillas
1 cup alfalfa sprouts

1. Place the chickpeas in a medium bowl, and mash until chunky.

2. Add celery, onion, grapes, yogurt, cashews, and curry powder, and stir until mixture is thoroughly combined.

3. Lay out tortillas on a clean work surface, and spread with filling, dividing evenly.

4. Top with the sprouts, and fold the tortillas to form tight pockets. Serve.

Serves 2   PREP TIME: 15 MINUTES
PER SERVING: CALORIES: 420 FAT: 10.5 GRAMS CHOLESTEROL: 1 MILLIGRAM
SODIUM: 360 MILLIGRAMS CARBOHYDRATES: 66.4 GRAMS
FIBER: 27.8 GRAMS PROTEIN: 29.4 GRAMS

Plan ahead for eating situations that may challenge your resolve. Your father-in-law wants to eat at the steak place that only has creamed spinach and au gratin potatoes as side dishes? Call the restaurant before you go to discuss your needs. Attending a children's birthday party where the only foods offered are pizza, cake, and soda? Call the host ahead of time and offer to bring a fruit salad or vegetable platter.

———————✳———————

Know your triggers. Keeping track of when and what you eat can help you figure out when you overeat or crave certain foods. Do you reach for a candy bar at 4 p.m.? Snack on chips just before dinner because you have not eaten anything since lunch? Once you know your triggers and eating patterns, you can take steps to change them.

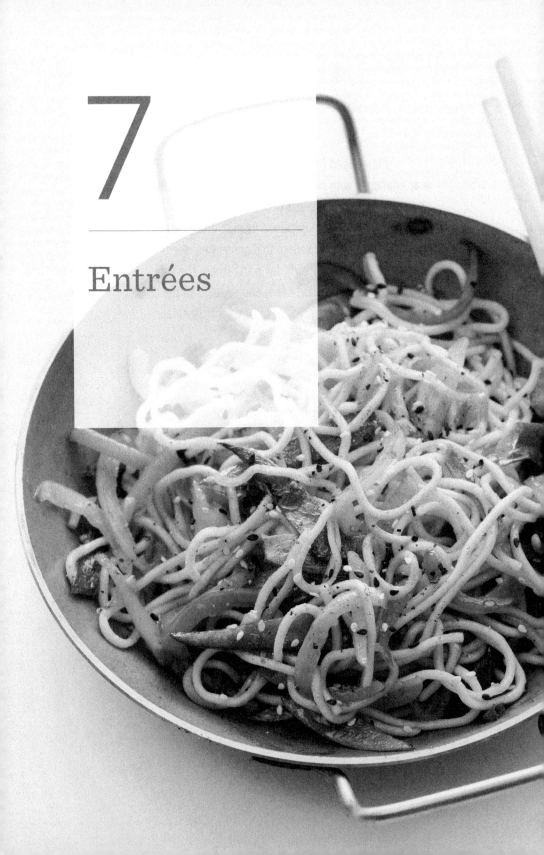

7

Entrées

RECIPES

Creamy Cheddar Grits with Shrimp

Arrowroot is a gluten-free substitute for wheat flour and has similar thickening properties when added to liquids. High in folate and other B vitamins, arrowroot is also a good source of potassium (454 milligrams per 100 grams, or 10 percent of RDA).

Grits

4 cups water

1 cup uncooked quick-cooking grits

$\frac{1}{2}$ cup shredded low-fat Cheddar cheese

$\frac{1}{4}$ teaspoon freshly ground pepper

Shrimp

1 pound medium-size raw shrimp, defrosted if frozen and peeled

$\frac{1}{4}$ teaspoon freshly ground pepper

2 tablespoons olive oil

2 garlic cloves, minced

$\frac{1}{2}$ cup snipped chives or scallions

$1\frac{1}{4}$ cups low-salt chicken broth

2 teaspoons arrowroot powder

1 tablespoon lemon juice

$\frac{1}{4}$ teaspoon smoked paprika

$\frac{1}{4}$ teaspoon hot sauce

1 tablespoon minced fresh tarragon

1. To prepare grits: In a medium saucepan, heat 4 cups water over high heat until boiling. Whisk in grits in a steady stream. Continue whisking to remove any lumps. Cover and cook over medium heat, stirring occasionally, for 8 minutes, or until thickened. Whisk in cheese and pepper, and turn off heat. Leave grits on stove, covered, to keep warm.

2. Sprinkle shrimp with pepper. Add 1 tablespoon of the olive oil to a large, nonstick sauté pan, and heat over medium-high heat. Add shrimp, garlic, and chives or scallions, and cook 1 minute on each side, or until shrimp start to turn pink. Remove shrimp from skillet and set aside.

3. Reduce heat to medium. Add 1 tablespoon oil to the same sauté pan and heat for 30 seconds. Add broth and arrowroot powder. Cook 2 to 3 minutes, or until thickened.

4. Stir in shrimp, lemon juice, paprika, and hot sauce. Cook 1 minute, until shrimp are warm.

5. Serve shrimp over grits, with tarragon sprinkled on top.

Serves 4   PREP TIME: 10 MINUTES / COOKING TIME: 15 MINUTES
PER SERVING: CALORIES: 130 FAT: 7.9 GRAMS CHOLESTEROL: 3 MILLIGRAMS
SODIUM: 201 MILLIGRAMS CARBOHYDRATES: 9.8 GRAMS
FIBER: 0.3 GRAM PROTEIN: 4.7 GRAMS

Fish Tacos

A few adjustments to this classic seaside dish make it ideal for DASH. To make it quickly, use leftover fish from another meal, or prepared fish from the deli counter. Serve with a fresh fruit and tomato salsa.

Guacamole

2 avocados, halved, pitted, and peeled

1 jalapeño, seeded and thinly sliced

2 tablespoons finely chopped red onion

2 tablespoons finely chopped cilantro

3 tablespoons lime juice

Freshly ground pepper to taste

Cabbage Slaw

½ head savoy cabbage, shredded (about 4 cups)

2 tablespoons olive oil

2 tablespoons lime juice

Freshly ground pepper to taste

Canola oil for brushing fish

1 pound wild Alaskan salmon, US-sourced yellowfin tuna, shrimp, or other healthy fish

Freshly ground pepper to taste

4 corn tortillas

2 tablespoons low-fat sour cream for serving

Hot sauce for serving

Lime wedges for serving

1. Light a grill unless using previously prepared fish.

2. To make guacamole: In a medium bowl, mash the avocados, jalapeño, red onion, cilantro, and lime juice. Season the guacamole with pepper. Set aside.

3. To make cabbage slaw: In a large bowl, toss the cabbage with the olive oil and the lime juice. Season with pepper. Set aside.

4. Brush the fish with canola oil, and season with pepper to taste. Grill over moderately high heat until lightly charred and cooked through, about 10 minutes for salmon or about 2 minutes for shrimp. Transfer the fish to a platter. (If using previously prepared, skip this step.)

5. While fish is cooking, warm tortillas according to package directions.

6. To assemble each taco, spread a dollop of guacamole on a tortilla. Top with a piece of fish and a large spoonful of the cabbage slaw. Serve with sour cream, hot sauce, and lime wedges.

Serves 4   PREP TIME: 15 MINUTES / COOKING TIME: 15 MINUTES
PER SERVING: CALORIES: 402 FAT: 24.2 GRAMS CHOLESTEROL: 67.5 MILLIGRAMS
SODIUM: 89.7 MILLIGRAMS CARBOHYDRATES: 13.9 GRAMS
FIBER: 8.9 GRAMS PROTEIN: 34.9 GRAMS

Tuna Salad Sandwiches

Usually loaded with high-fat mayonnaise, tuna salad does not often come to mind as a healthful staple. This version is made with Greek yogurt and flavorful roasted peppers, adding taste and moisture without a lot of fat. Roasted red bell peppers are available by the jar and at many supermarket salad and olive bars and are a good low-salt option.

One 6-ounce can low-salt albacore or skipjack white tuna,
    packed in water, drained
1 slice roasted red bell pepper from a jar, drained and finely chopped
4 artichoke heart halves from a can or jar, drained and
    finely chopped
½ red onion, finely chopped
¼ cup plain nonfat Greek-style yogurt
1 tablespoon dried oregano
Juice of 1 lemon
Freshly ground pepper to taste
1 cup mixed greens
4 slices quinoa and millet or spelt bread

1. In a small bowl, combine tuna, red pepper, artichokes, onion, yogurt, oregano, and lemon juice and mix well. Season with pepper to taste.

2. Toast or warm the bread.

3. Layer the greens on the bread, then top with the tuna salad. Serve immediately.

Serves 2   PREP TIME: 10 MINUTES
PER SERVING: CALORIES: 327 FAT: 6.5 GRAMS CHOLESTEROL: 15 MILLIGRAMS
SODIUM: 389 MILLIGRAMS CARBOHYDRATES: 52.6 GRAMS
FIBER: 7.6 GRAMS PROTEIN: 22.1 GRAMS

Grilled Halibut with Spiced Yogurt

Using a cast-iron skillet eliminates the difficulty of moving fish around the grill. If halibut isn't available, this recipe works equally well with salmon or just about any sturdy fish.

1 teaspoon honey

1 teaspoon low-salt soy sauce

1 teaspoon fresh minced ginger

1 teaspoon sesame oil

Two 6-ounce halibut fillets

1 tablespoon olive oil

$\frac{1}{2}$ teaspoon sambal oelek or garlic chili sauce

One 6-ounce container plain nonfat Greek-style yogurt

1. Preheat grill to high. Place a cast-iron skillet on the grill to warm.

2. In a pie pan, swirl together the honey, soy sauce, ginger, and sesame oil. Place halibut fillets, skin side up, in the pan. Marinate for 15 minutes. ➤

Grilled Halibut with Spicy Yogurt *continued*

3. Add olive oil to the cast-iron pan, and swirl to coat. Add fish, skin-side up, and sear for 1 minute. Flip fish over, reduce heat to medium, and cook fish an additional 6 minutes. Remove from the heat.

4. In a small bowl, mix together the sambal oelek or garlic chili sauce and yogurt. Serve with the fish.

Serves 2   PREP TIME: 20 MINUTES / COOKING TIME: 10 MINUTES
PER SERVING: CALORIES: 285 FAT: 5.6 GRAMS CHOLESTEROL: 69.7 MILLIGRAMS
SODIUM: 346.1 MILLIGRAMS CARBOHYDRATES: 3.3 GRAMS
FIBER: 0 GRAMS PROTEIN: 53 GRAMS

Black-Eyed Pea Burgers

Mushrooms are moist, tender, and loaded with umami, *which is a Japanese word for the savory basic taste intrinsic to certain foods. The addition of umami-rich foods lends a pleasant meatiness to vegetarian and non-vegetarian dishes alike. These rich, tasty burgers are loaded with micronutrients and iron. Try them without bread—you may find them filling enough on their own—or add a lettuce wrap to boost your vegetable servings for the day.*

5 tablespoons grape seed or olive oil

4 ounces cremini mushrooms, cleaned, stemmed, and
    cut into $\frac{1}{4}$-inch thick slices

$\frac{1}{4}$ teaspoon dried thyme

2 garlic cloves, minced

$\frac{1}{2}$ chopped red onion, plus more for serving

One 15-ounce can low-salt black-eyed peas, drained and rinsed

2 tablespoons fresh basil or parsley, minced

$\frac{1}{2}$ teaspoon wheat-free tamari

4 large lettuce leaves or spelt bread

1 avocado, sliced

1. Heat 3 tablespoons of the oil in a large frying pan over medium heat until shimmering. Add the mushrooms and thyme. Cook, stirring occasionally, until browned, about 2 to 3 minutes. Add the garlic and red onion, and cook until fragrant and softened, about 2 minutes. Remove from heat.

2. Place the black-eyed peas in a large bowl, and mash with the back of a spoon or a potato masher, leaving a few of the peas intact. Add the mushroom mixture, basil or parsley, and tamari, and mix until combined. Form the mixture into four patties. ➤

Black-Eyed Pea Burgers *continued*

3. Heat the remaining 2 tablespoons oil in a sauté pan over medium-high heat until shimmering. Add the patties and fry until browned, about 5 to 6 minutes per side.

4. Serve on bread or lettuce leaves with additional red onion and avocado.

Serves 4   PREP TIME: 10 MINUTES / COOKING TIME: 15 MINUTES
PER SERVING: CALORIES: 317 FAT: 25.4 GRAMS CHOLESTEROL: 0 MILLIGRAMS
SODIUM: 51.7 MILLIGRAMS CARBOHYDRATES: 22.5 GRAMS
FIBER: 7.6 GRAMS PROTEIN: 4.2 GRAMS

Bean and Vegetable Tacos

This recipe works equally well with shrimp or leftover cooked chicken in place of the black beans.

3 tablespoons olive oil

One 1-pound package pre-cut stir-fry vegetables

One 15-ounce can low-salt black beans, drained and rinsed

1 teaspoon dried oregano

$1\frac{1}{2}$ tablespoons lime juice

$\frac{1}{2}$ teaspoon hot sauce

4 corn tortillas

$\frac{1}{2}$ cup (2 ounces) shredded Mexican cheese blend

1 avocado, sliced

$\frac{1}{2}$ cup chopped tomato

1. Heat 2 tablespoons of the oil in a large sauté pan over medium heat. Add stir-fry vegetables to pan, and cook until vegetables have softened, 6 to 8 minutes. Remove from heat.

2. In a medium bowl, combine beans, oregano, lime juice, hot sauce, and remaining tablespoon olive oil.

3. Warm tortillas according to package directions.

4. Top each tortilla with bean mixture, cheese, avocado, and chopped tomato. Serve.

Serves 4   PREP TIME: 15 MINUTES / COOKING TIME: 8 MINUTES
PER SERVING: CALORIES: 409 FAT: 21.3 GRAMS CHOLESTEROL: 6.3 MILLIGRAMS
SODIUM: 90.4 MILLIGRAMS CARBOHYDRATES: 44.3 GRAMS
FIBER: 14.5 GRAMS PROTEIN: 14.9 GRAMS

Turkey Lettuce Cups

Wrapping this Asian-influenced ground turkey mixture in lettuce leaves instead of serving it with bread reduces carbs and increases your vegetable intake.

2 teaspoons sesame oil

1¼ pounds lean ground turkey

1 tablespoon minced ginger (fresh or jarred)

One 12-ounce can baby corn, drained and chopped into 1-inch pieces

One 8-ounce can water chestnuts, drained and chopped

4 scallions, minced

1 cup 1-inch pieces snap peas

½ cup low-salt chicken broth

2 tablespoons hoisin sauce

8 leaves Bibb lettuce

½ cup chopped fresh cilantro

1 carrot, shredded

1. Heat oil in a large nonstick pan over medium-high heat. Add turkey and ginger and cook, crumbling with a wooden spoon, until the turkey is cooked through, about 8 minutes.

2. Stir in the baby corn, water chestnuts, scallions, snap peas, broth, and hoisin sauce. Cook 1 more minute.

3. Spoon some of the turkey mixture into each lettuce leaf, top with cilantro and carrot, and roll into wraps. Serve immediately.

Serves 4   PREP TIME: 15 MINUTES / COOKING TIME: 10 MINUTES
PER SERVING: CALORIES: 275 FAT: 12.6 GRAMS CHOLESTEROL: 29 MILLIGRAMS
SODIUM: 296 MILLIGRAMS CARBOHYDRATES: 9.5 GRAMS
FIBER: 1.5 GRAMS PROTEIN: 28.8 GRAMS

Turkey Sloppy Joes

Kids of all ages will enjoy this reduced-fat, low-sodium version of a classic American sandwich. Curry powder adds healthy flavor—you won't miss the canned or bottled chili sauce. If you happen to have tomato jam, you can use it in place of the tomato sauce for added tang.

2 teaspoons canola oil

1 onion, chopped

1 ¼ pound lean ground turkey

1 teaspoon curry powder

½ cup low-salt tomato sauce or tomato jam

4 spelt buns

1 cup baby spinach leaves

½ cup plain low-fat yogurt

1. In a medium nonstick sauté pan, heat oil over medium heat. Add onion and cook until translucent, about 6 minutes. Add turkey and cook, crumbling with a spoon, until turkey is cooked through, about 8 minutes.

2. Add curry powder and cook until fragrant, about 30 seconds. Add tomato sauce or tomato jam, and cook until heated through, about 2 minutes.

3. Remove from heat. Serve on buns topped with spinach leaves and drizzled with yogurt.

Serves 4   PREP TIME: 15 MINUTES / COOKING TIME: 8 MINUTES
PER SERVING: CALORIES: 447 FAT: 15.3 GRAMS CHOLESTEROL: 29 MILLIGRAMS
SODIUM: 297.4 MILLIGRAMS CARBOHYDRATES: 42.4 GRAMS
FIBER: 3.4 GRAMS PROTEIN: 35.2 GRAMS

Chicken Dippers with Peanut Sauce

If you can't find low-salt fish sauce, leave it out and add another tea-spoon of low-salt soy sauce. (Caution: People with shellfish allergies are sensitive to fish sauce.)

3 tablespoons lime juice
3 tablespoons canola oil
3 teaspoons low-salt soy sauce
2 teaspoons honey
$\frac{1}{4}$ teaspoon cayenne pepper
1 pound boneless chicken strips

Peanut Sauce
2 tablespoons smooth peanut butter
2 tablespoons low-fat coconut milk
1 tablespoon lime juice
1 teaspoon low-salt fish sauce

1. Preheat a grill. In a pie plate, whisk together lime juice, oil, 2 teaspoons soy sauce, honey, and cayenne. Add the chicken and turn to coat. Let marinate 15 minutes.

2. To make peanut sauce: In a medium bowl, whisk together peanut butter, coconut milk, lime juice, fish sauce, and 1 teaspoon soy sauce. Set aside.

3. Grill chicken until cooked through, about 3 minutes per side. Serve with peanut sauce.

Serves 4   PREP TIME: 15 MINUTES / COOKING TIME: 8 MINUTES
PER SERVING: CALORIES: 204 FAT: 8.9 GRAMS CHOLESTEROL: 70.2 MILLIGRAMS
SODIUM: 175.3 MILLIGRAMS CARBOHYDRATES: 2.2 GRAMS
FIBER: 0.8 GRAM PROTEIN: 28 GRAMS

Pork Loin with Figgy Sauce

Pork loin is a lean meat and pairs beautifully with figs. To change up the recipe, reduce the figs to ½ cup and add ½ cup dried apricots. This dish is perfect for entertaining.

2 teaspoons dried rosemary

1 teaspoon dried thyme

½ teaspoon freshly ground pepper

Two 1¼-pound pork loins

¼ cup olive oil

3 carrots, peeled and cut on the diagonal into ½-inch pieces

1 onion, chopped

3 garlic cloves, minced

1 cup dried figs, cut into quarters

1 cup white wine

Juice of 1 lemon

1. Preheat the oven to 350°F. In a small bowl, mix the rosemary, thyme, and pepper to make a spice rub, and press into the pork loins.

2. Heat the olive oil over medium heat in a large, oven-proof skillet. Add the pork loin, carrots, onion, and garlic, and cook for 4 minutes per side. ➤

Pork Loin with Figgy Sauce *continued*

3. Add the figs, white wine, and lemon juice to the skillet. Remove from heat. Cover with aluminum foil, and bake in the oven for 20 to 30 minutes, or until the internal temperature of the pork is about 145°F. Transfer the meat to a cutting board, and tent with aluminum foil.

4. While pork is resting, transfer the vegetables, figs, and pan juices into a blender. Process until smooth to make a gravy. Serve gravy with the pork.

Serves 8   PREP TIME: 15 MINUTES / COOKING TIME: 30 TO 40 MINUTES
PER SERVING: CALORIES: 386 FAT: 14.3 GRAMS CHOLESTEROL: 60 MILLIGRAMS
SODIUM: 79 MILLIGRAMS CARBOHYDRATES: 27 GRAMS
FIBER: 4.1 GRAMS PROTEIN: 36 GRAMS

Buffalo Burgers

Buffalo is a lean red meat, raised from start to finish on grass. It is never fed corn or byproducts, so its meat has a clean, fresh flavor. Because buffalo is low in fat, it cooks more quickly than conventional beef burgers. Grill at medium heat.

1 pound ground buffalo (American bison) meat
1 teaspoon freshly ground pepper
1 teaspoon smoked paprika
$\frac{1}{2}$ yellow onion, minced
$\frac{1}{4}$ cup smoky barbecue sauce such as chipotle-honey,
    plus more for serving
8 slices spelt bread or 4 spelt buns
4 slices smoked low-fat mozzarella cheese

1. Preheat grill to medium. In a large bowl, combine buffalo meat, pepper, paprika, minced onion, and barbecue sauce until well mixed. Shape into four patties.

2. Place patties on the grill, and sear for about 3 minutes per side, or until cooked through.

3. Serve on spelt bread or buns topped with cheese and additional barbecue sauce.

Serves 4   PREP TIME: 15 MINUTES / COOKING TIME: 8 MINUTES
PER SERVING: CALORIES: 512 FAT: 24.1 GRAMS CHOLESTEROL: 72 MILLIGRAMS
SODIUM: 425 MILLIGRAMS CARBOHYDRATES: 35 GRAMS
FIBER: 2.2 GRAMS PROTEIN: 42 GRAMS

Grilled Skirt Steak with Salsa Verde

Skirt steak is lean, flavorful, and not too pricey. To serve, slice it across the grain to ensure tenderness.

One 1½-pound skirt steak
½ teaspoon freshly ground pepper
¼ cup grape seed oil
Zest of 1 lemon
2 garlic cloves, minced

Salsa Verde
¼ cup olive oil
1 cup minced soft herbs such as fresh mint, tarragon, or basil
1 cup minced fresh parsley
2 avocados, cut into ¼-inch dice
1 cup plain low-fat Greek yogurt

1. Preheat grill. In a large bowl, sprinkle steak with pepper. Add grape seed oil, lemon zest, and garlic, and stir to combine. Allow to marinate for 20 minutes.

2. To make salsa verde: In a medium bowl, toss olive oil with herbs and parsley. Stir in avocado. Stir in yogurt, ¼ cup at a time, until the salsa reaches a consistency you like.

3. Grill steak until charred, about 2 minutes per side for medium-rare. Allow to rest before slicing. Serve with salsa.

Serves 4   PREP TIME: 20 MINUTES / COOKING TIME: 5 MINUTES
PER SERVING: CALORIES: 684 FAT: 56.7 GRAMS CHOLESTEROL: 87.5 MILLIGRAMS
SODIUM: 116.7 MILLIGRAMS CARBOHYDRATES: 12.8 GRAMS
FIBER: 7.8 GRAMS PROTEIN: 33 GRAMS

Lamb Kebabs with Garlic and Mint

Lamb is a lean, quick-cooking meat. Anchovies are loaded with heart-healthy fatty acids and add an astringent contrast to the rich taste of lamb. Serve with a side of Cannellini Bean Salad with Mint and Parsley (recipe on page 115) and a green salad.

2 anchovies
2 garlic cloves, minced
3 tablespoons plus ¼ cup olive oil
2 pounds lamb leg, cut into 2-inch cubes
¼ cup chopped fresh mint

1. In a medium bowl, mash together the anchovies and garlic until a coarse paste forms. Add 3 tablespoons of the olive oil and the lamb, and mix until the lamb is evenly coated. Let mixture rest for 15 minutes or up to 2 hours.

2. Light a grill and heat to medium-high. Thread lamb cubes onto metal skewers. When the grill is hot, sear the lamb to medium-rare, about 5 minutes per side.

3. Meanwhile, mix remaining olive oil and mint in a small bowl.

4. Place the lamb kebabs on serving tray, and sprinkle with mint oil to serve.

Serves 6   PREP TIME: 5 MINUTES / COOKING TIME: 15 MINUTES
PER SERVING: CALORIES: 227 FAT: 10.3 GRAMS CHOLESTEROL: 97.9 MILLIGRAMS
SODIUM: 171 MILLIGRAMS CARBOHYDRATES: 0 GRAMS
FIBER: 0 GRAMS PROTEIN: 31.3 GRAMS

Broiled Curried Chicken and Yogurt Tenders

This dish is perfect for a busy evening, because it can go from fridge to table in less than 30 minutes. Serve the chicken with steamed brown rice and asparagus tips for a balanced DASH diet meal. Broiling is a tasty cooking method that will not add any extra calories to the chicken.

$^3/_4$ cup plain fat-free yogurt

Juice of 1 lemon

1 tablespoon curry powder

1 teaspoon minced garlic

$^1/_4$ teaspoon freshly ground pepper

Four 5-ounce boneless, skinless chicken breasts, each cut
    into 4 thin strips

1 tablespoon chopped fresh cilantro

1. Line a baking sheet with foil.

2. Whisk yogurt, lemon juice, curry powder, garlic, and pepper together in a small bowl until well blended.

3. Place chicken strips in a sealable plastic bag, and add yogurt mixture. Squeeze bag to coat chicken evenly. Place chicken in fridge for 30 minutes.

4. Preheat oven to broil. Place top oven rack about 6 inches from broiler heat.

5. Spread chicken in prepared baking sheet.

6. Place chicken under broiler, and broil until chicken is cooked through, turning once, about 20 minutes.

7. Serve hot with brown rice, and sprinkle with fresh cilantro.

Serves 4   PREP TIME: 5 MINUTES / COOKING TIME: 20 MINUTES
PER SERVING: CALORIES: 286 FAT: 10.5 GRAMS CHOLESTEROL: 127 MILLIGRAMS
SODIUM: 148 MILLIGRAMS CARBOHYDRATES: 2.9 GRAMS
FIBER: 0.6 GRAM PROTEIN: 42.6 GRAMS

Wild Rice and Chicken-Stuffed Tomatoes

If you want to add a little extra flavor to this dish, you can cook the wild rice in low-sodium chicken or vegetable stock. Make sure you read the label on the stock carefully because some reduced-sodium products still contain a large amount of salt. Use 2 cups stock to 1 cup rice for the best results. For a vegetarian version of the recipe, replace the chicken with one 16-ounce can of low-salt chickpeas or lentils.

4 large tomatoes

2 cups cooked wild rice

One 8-ounce cooked boneless, skinless chicken breast, chopped

1 celery stalk, finely chopped

2 teaspoons minced garlic

$\frac{1}{2}$ cup grated Parmesan cheese

$\frac{1}{4}$ cup chopped unsalted pistachios

4 teaspoons chopped fresh basil

2 teaspoons olive oil

Freshly ground pepper

1. Preheat oven to 350°F.

2. Carefully cut tops off tomatoes and scoop out with a spoon, leaving an intact shell and reserving interior pulp. Place shells in a shallow baking dish.

3. Chop reserved tomato pulp coarsely and transfer to a medium bowl.

4. Add cooked rice, chicken, celery, garlic, cheese, pistachios, and basil to the tomato pulp, and mix well.

5. Spoon filling evenly into tomato shells. Drizzle each prepared tomato with olive oil.

6. Bake stuffed tomatoes in oven until filling is piping hot and tomatoes are softened but not collapsed, about 20 minutes.

7. Season with pepper and serve with a salad.

Serves 4   PREP TIME: 15 MINUTES / COOKING TIME: 20 MINUTES
PER SERVING: CALORIES: 503 FAT: 11.8 GRAMS CHOLESTEROL: 47 MILLIGRAMS
SODIUM: 243 MILLIGRAMS CARBOHYDRATES: 70.4 GRAMS
FIBER: 8.1 GRAMS PROTEIN: 33.6 GRAMS

Ratatouille with Pasta

Eating plenty of vegetables is a great strategy for general good health and goes a long way in meeting DASH goals. This Mediterranean-inspired pasta dish is bursting with flavor and nutritious, colorful produce. You can also serve the ratatouille with brown rice instead of pasta, or eat it plain as a stew.

1 tablespoon olive oil

1 large sweet onion, chopped

3 teaspoons minced garlic

1 small eggplant, cut into $\frac{1}{2}$-inch cubes

2 small green zucchini, diced

1 red bell pepper, seeded and diced

2 large tomatoes, diced

$\frac{1}{2}$ teaspoon freshly ground pepper

Pinch of red pepper flakes

2 tablespoons chopped fresh basil

6 cups multigrain spaghetti, cooked according to
   package instructions

1. Heat olive oil in a large skillet over medium-high heat.

2. Add onion and garlic and sauté until tender, about 4 minutes.

3. Add eggplant, zucchini, and bell pepper. Sauté until softened, about 10 minutes.

4. Add tomato, pepper, and red pepper flakes.

5. Continue to cook, stirring occasionally, until vegetables are tender and liquid reduces to a sauce texture, about 7 minutes.

6. Stir in basil and cooked pasta, and cook until pasta is warmed through, stirring occasionally, about 4 minutes. Serve hot.

Serves 6   PREP TIME: 10 MINUTES / COOKING TIME: 25 MINUTES
PER SERVING: CALORIES: 394 FAT: 4.7 GRAMS CHOLESTEROL: 0 MILLIGRAMS
SODIUM: 9 MILLIGRAMS CARBOHYDRATES: 73.9 GRAMS
FIBER: 14.7 GRAMS PROTEIN: 14.1 GRAMS

Speedy Turkey Chili

You can use any combination of beans in this hearty dish, depending on your preference. Black-eyed peas, lentils, pinto beans, white kidney beans, and split peas also work very well with the seasonings. If you cannot find good-quality low-salt products, you can rehydrate dry beans—which saves you money as well as allowing you to control the salt level. Simply follow the package instructions, and your dish will be perfect.

1 teaspoon olive oil

½ pound lean ground turkey

1 small sweet onion, chopped

1 teaspoon minced garlic

One 16-ounce can low-salt red kidney beans, rinsed and drained

One 16-ounce can low-salt chickpeas, rinsed and drained

One 16-ounce can low-salt navy beans, rinsed and drained

One 16-ounce can low-salt black beans, rinsed and drained

4 large tomatoes, diced

3 tablespoons chili powder

1 teaspoon ground cumin

1. In a large pot over medium-high heat, add olive oil. Sauté turkey meat in oil until completely cooked through, about 6 minutes.

2. Add onion and garlic and cook, stirring frequently, until translucent, about 3 minutes.

3. Add kidney beans, chickpeas, navy beans, black beans, tomatoes, chili powder, and cumin. Bring to a boil, then reduce heat to a simmer. Simmer, stirring occasionally, for 20 to 25 minutes.

4. Remove from heat and serve hot.

Serves 6   PREP TIME: 5 MINUTES / COOKING TIME: 35 MINUTES
PER SERVING: CALORIES: 383 FAT: 6.1 GRAMS CHOLESTEROL: 27 MILLIGRAMS
SODIUM: 109 MILLIGRAMS CARBOHYDRATES: 55.5 GRAMS
FIBER: 21.9 GRAMS PROTEIN: 28.6 GRAMS

Pork Tenderloin with Herbes de Provence

Herbes de Provence might sound like a lofty ingredient, but it is simply a mixture of herbs usually used in French cooking, including thyme, rosemary, savory, oregano, and marjoram. Other herbs are included in these mixes as well, depending on the brand and area where it was made. It sometimes even contains lavender. You can mix up your own combination using fresh and dried herbs if you want a custom flavor profile for this dish.

16 ounces pork tenderloin, trimmed of fat and cut
   crosswise into 8 pieces
Freshly ground pepper
1 tablespoon olive oil
1 tablespoon herbes de Provence
$\frac{1}{2}$ cup low-salt chicken stock or white wine

1. Place pork pieces between pieces of parchment paper. Using a mallet or the flat side of a meat tenderizer, pound each piece to about $\frac{1}{4}$ inch thick.

2. Season pork lightly with pepper on both sides.

3. Place a large skillet over medium-high heat, and add olive oil.

4. Fry pork until just cooked through and lightly browned, about 2 minutes per side.

5. Remove pork, and keep warm on a foil-covered plate.

6. Return skillet to heat, and pour in stock or wine.

7. Bring mixture to a boil, and with a wooden spoon, scrape up flavorful browned bits from bottom of skillet. Reduce heat to low and simmer until sauce reduces a little and thickens slightly, about 2 minutes.

8. Add the herbes de Provence and pork juices that have accumulated on plate.

9. Remove sauce from heat. Serve pork hot, with sauce.

Serves 4   PREP TIME: 5 MINUTES / COOKING TIME: 10 MINUTES
PER SERVING: CALORIES: 187 FAT: 4 GRAMS CHOLESTEROL: 83 MILLIGRAMS
SODIUM: 66 MILLIGRAMS CARBOHYDRATES: 0.8 GRAM
FIBER: 1.4 GRAMS PROTEIN: 29.7 GRAMS

Spicy Chinese Noodles

Stir-frying is one of the healthier techniques for cooking. It uses minimal fat, and the food is usually not drenched in sodium-laced sauces. You can add a teaspoon of low-sodium soy sauce to this dish without going outside of DASH recommendations, but these noodles are delicious without the addition.

One 8-ounce package Chinese rice noodles

1 tablespoon sesame oil

1 tablespoon minced garlic

1 tablespoon grated peeled fresh ginger

2 green onions, sliced thinly

2 medium carrots, peeled and sliced thinly into disks

1 cup small broccoli florets

1 cup sliced mushrooms

1 cup halved snow peas, strings removed

1 cup fresh bean sprouts

1 gently packed cup shredded fresh spinach

Red pepper flakes

$\frac{1}{4}$ cup chopped roasted almonds

1. Cook rice noodles according to package instructions. Drain and set aside.

2. Place a large skillet over medium-high heat, and add sesame oil.

3. Sauté ginger and garlic until softened, about 3 minutes.

4. Add green onions, reserving 2 tablespoons, and sauté until softened, about 1 minute.

5. Add carrots and broccoli, and stir-fry until vegetables are crisp-tender, about 4 minutes.

6. Add mushrooms and snow peas, and stir-fry, about 2 minutes.

7. Stir in bean sprouts and spinach, and stir-fry until spinach is wilted, about 2 minutes or less.

8. Remove pan from heat, and stir in red pepper flakes.

9. Toss rice noodles with vegetables until well combined.

10. Serve hot, topped with chopped almonds and reserved green onion.

Serves 4   PREP TIME: 20 MINUTES / COOKING TIME: 12 MINUTES
PER SERVING: CALORIES: 150 FAT: 6.8 GRAMS CHOLESTEROL: 0 MILLIGRAMS
SODIUM: 40 MILLIGRAMS CARBOHYDRATES: 17.9 GRAMS
FIBER: 5.7 GRAMS PROTEIN: 8.2 GRAMS

Vegetarian Kebabs

If you have a barbecue, these kebabs are delicious grilled over medium heat. You can use any combination of vegetables on the skewer, such as baby portobello mushrooms, red or yellow bell peppers, sweet potato chunks, or eggplant. Get a nice assortment of colors so you get a broad range of phytonutrients on your plate. Serve with rice.

4 tablespoons olive oil
2 tablespoons balsamic vinegar
1 teaspoon minced garlic
$\frac{1}{2}$ teaspoon chopped fresh thyme
$\frac{1}{2}$ teaspoon chopped fresh oregano
Freshly ground pepper
2 small zucchini, cut into 16 chunks
2 small white or red onions, peeled and cut into quarters
16 cherry tomatoes
16 medium button mushrooms
1 cup broccoli florets
2 red, yellow, or green bell peppers, seeded and cut into 8 slices each
8 wooden skewers, soaked in water for 30 minutes

1. In a small bowl, whisk together olive oil, vinegar, garlic, thyme, oregano, and pepper.

2. Pour marinade into a large zipper-top plastic bag, and add zucchini, onions, tomatoes, mushrooms, and bell peppers.

3. Shake to coat, and place in fridge for at least 30 minutes.

4. Preheat oven to broil, and place an oven rack about 6 inches from broiler heat.

5. Take marinating vegetables out of fridge, and thread onto skewers, dividing evenly. On each skewer, place 2 zucchini pieces, 1 piece of onion, 2 tomatoes, 2 mushrooms, and 2 pieces of bell pepper.

6. Pour remaining marinade in a small bowl to baste vegetables.

7. Place skewers on a baking sheet or oven grill rack, and broil, turning once and basting with reserved marinade, until vegetables are tender, about 10 minutes. Serve hot.

Serves 4   PREP TIME: 15 MINUTES / COOKING TIME: 10 MINUTES
PER SERVING: CALORIES: 210 FAT: 8.5 GRAMS CHOLESTEROL: 0 MILLIGRAMS
SODIUM: 37 MILLIGRAMS CARBOHYDRATES: 30.9 GRAMS
FIBER: 9.5 GRAMS PROTEIN: 8.3 GRAMS

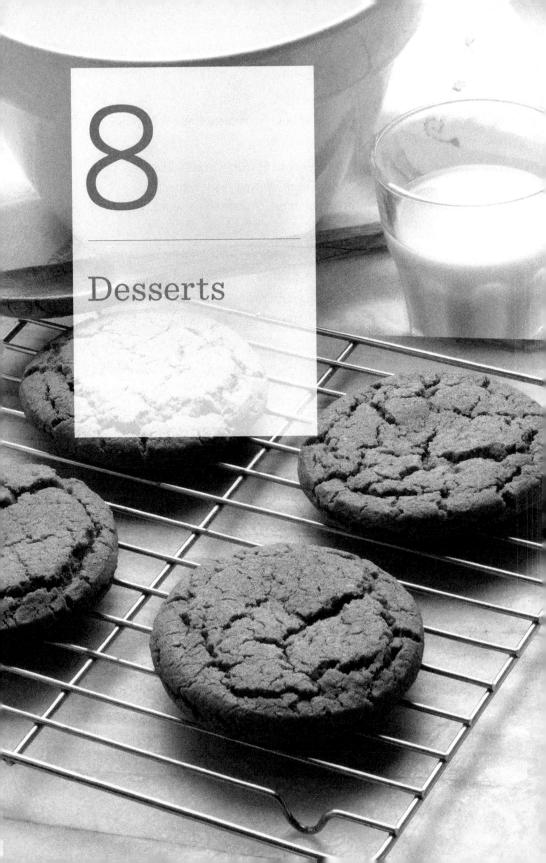

8

Desserts

RECIPES

Lightened Whipped Cream

Evaporated milk has a deeper, richer flavor than cream or skim milk. If the flavor of the whipped cream is too heavy for the dessert you have planned, try adding a tablespoon of prepared mocha coffee or cocoa powder when you add the sugar, or fold in a tablespoon of crystallized ginger just before serving. A serving is 1 tablespoon of whipped cream.

⅓ cup evaporated nonfat milk, chilled
2 tablespoons granulated sugar
2 tablespoons plain low-fat yogurt

1. Pour milk into a deep mixing bowl, and place in the freezer for 30 minutes.

2. Remove bowl from freezer and whip with an electric mixer at high speed until the milk is the consistency of fluffy whipped cream, 1 to 2 minutes.

3. Add sugar and yogurt, and whip until thickened, 3 minutes. Serve immediately.

Serves 16   PREP TIME: 35 MINUTES
PER SERVING: CALORIES: 20 FAT: 0 GRAMS CHOLESTEROL: 0 MILLIGRAMS
SODIUM: 7 MILLIGRAMS CARBOHYDRATES: 4 GRAMS
FIBER: 0 GRAMS PROTEIN: 0 GRAMS

Fruit Kebabs

This pretty, healthful, and fun variation on fruit salad gets a spicy kick from ginger and cayenne pepper.

3 tablespoons lime juice

3 tablespoons orange juice

1 tablespoon jarred minced ginger

¾ cup cantaloupe chunks

¾ cup star fruit, cut into ½-inch slices

¾ cup strawberries

¾ cup peach chunks

One 6-ounce container nonfat vanilla yogurt

⅛ teaspoon cayenne pepper

1. In a shallow lasagna pan, combine lime juice, orange juice, and ginger.

2. Thread cantaloupe, star fruit, strawberries, and peaches onto eight skewers. Arrange on top of juice mixture and turn to coat.

3. In a small bowl, combine yogurt and cayenne.

4. Remove skewers from marinade, and serve with spiced yogurt.

Serves 8   PREP TIME: 15 MINUTES
PER SERVING: CALORIES: 91 FAT: 1 GRAM CHOLESTEROL: 2 MILLIGRAMS
SODIUM: 20 MILLIGRAMS CARBOHYDRATES: 21 GRAMS
FIBER: 1 GRAM PROTEIN: 2 GRAMS

Pumpkin Seed Brittle

Pumpkin seeds are a good source of magnesium. This brittle, wrapped in a bow, makes a lovely gift.

$\frac{1}{2}$ teaspoon cayenne pepper
$\frac{1}{4}$ teaspoon grated nutmeg
1 cup roasted, unsalted pumpkin seeds
1 cup granulated stevia
$\frac{1}{2}$ cup granulated sugar
$\frac{1}{4}$ cup water

1. Line a jelly roll pan with parchment paper or a baking mat. Combine cayenne, nutmeg, and pumpkin seeds in a small bowl and set aside.

2. In a large sauté pan, combine the stevia, sugar, and water, and cook over high heat, stirring constantly with a silicone spatula, until the mixture begins to boil, about 6 minutes. Using a pastry brush, swab down sides of pan so all sugar cooks evenly. Cook 3 more minutes without stirring.

3. Reduce heat to medium. Cook for another 15 to 20 minutes, checking frequently, until the mixture turns a golden, light brown color. Remove from heat.

4. Using a silicone spatula, quickly stir the pumpkin seed mixture into the sugar mixture. Pour into the prepared baking pan, and press firmly with the spatula to make a single, even layer.

5. Cool completely, then break into pieces and serve.

Serves 10   PREP TIME: 5 MINUTES / COOKING TIME: 25 MINUTES
PER SERVING: CALORIES: 20 FAT: 0 GRAMS CHOLESTEROL: 0 MILLIGRAMS
SODIUM: 7 MILLIGRAMS CARBOHYDRATES: 4 GRAMS
FIBER: 0 GRAMS PROTEIN: 0 GRAMS

Chocolate Pudding

Arrowroot is a good source of potassium, and cocoa is a good source of magnesium. Make this with calcium-fortified evaporated skim milk or other calcium-fortified milk to hit the DASH trifecta.

2 tablespoons unsweetened cocoa powder

½ tablespoon arrowroot powder

1 cup evaporated skim milk

2 tablespoons agave nectar or brown rice syrup

1 teaspoon vanilla extract

4 tablespoons roasted slivered almonds

1. In a medium nonstick pan, whisk together the cocoa powder and arrowroot powder.

2. Over medium heat, add evaporated skim milk and agave nectar to cocoa powder mixture, and whisk to combine. Bring just to a simmer, whisking constantly to make sure it does not boil.

3. Cook 3 to 5 minutes, or until pudding is thick. Remove from heat. Stir in vanilla.

4. Allow to rest 30 minutes before serving or chill overnight. Spoon into four bowls. Top each bowl with 1 tablespoon of the almonds, and serve.

Serves 4   PREP TIME: 5 MINUTES / COOKING TIME: 15 MINUTES
PER SERVING: CALORIES: 89 FAT: 3.7 GRAMS CHOLESTEROL: 0 MILLIGRAMS
SODIUM: 60.3 MILLIGRAMS CARBOHYDRATES: 11.5 GRAMS
FIBER: 1.4 GRAMS PROTEIN: 5.8 GRAMS

Fudgy Sauce

Blackstrap molasses is a good source of calcium. Here it adds a rich flavor to the sauce.

2 tablespoons unsweetened cocoa powder

1 teaspoon instant coffee

1 teaspoon arrowroot powder

½ cup evaporated skim milk

¼ cup blackstrap molassas

1. In a small nonstick sauté pan, stir together the cocoa, instant coffee, and arrowroot powder. Whisk in the milk; then the molasses.

2. Place the pan over medium heat. Cook, stirring constantly, until the sauce is smooth and thickened, 5 to 10 minutes. Remove from heat, and allow sauce to cool 4 minutes before serving.

Serves 8 PREP TIME: 5 MINUTES / COOKING TIME: 10 MINUTES
PER SERVING: CALORIES: 39 FAT: 0.3 GRAM CHOLESTEROL: 0 MILLIGRAMS
SODIUM: 20.9 MILLIGRAMS CARBOHYDRATES: 9.4 GRAMS
FIBER: 0.7 GRAM PROTEIN: 1.4 GRAMS

Figs with Chocolate Sauce

Figs are often overlooked as a source of nutrients, but ¼ cup of dried figs contains 75 milligrams of calcium.

8 fresh or dried figs
¼ cup honey
2 tablespoons unsweetened cocoa powder
½ cup plain low-fat Greek-style yogurt

1. If using dried figs, place the figs in a small heat-proof bowl. Add boiling water to cover. Let rest in the hot water for 5 to 15 minutes; then drain before continuing.

2. Combine the honey and cocoa powder in a small bowl, and mix well to form a syrup.

3. Cut the figs in half and place cut side up. Drizzle with the syrup, top with a dollop of yogurt, and serve.

Serves 4   PREP TIME: 5 MINUTES / COOKING TIME: 10 MINUTES
PER SERVING: CALORIES: 142.6 FAT: 0.6 GRAM CHOLESTEROL: 0 MILLIGRAMS
SODIUM: 12.2 MILLIGRAMS CARBOHYDRATES: 35.1 GRAMS
FIBER: 3.3 GRAMS PROTEIN: 3.7 GRAMS

Berries with Balsamic Vinegar and Black Pepper

Balsamic vinegar and black pepper add a surprising zip to the berries in this dish.

¼ cup balsamic vinegar
1 tablespoon brown sugar
¼ teaspoon freshly ground pepper
½ cup sliced strawberries
½ cup blueberries
½ cup raspberries
4 tablespoons plain, unsweetened low-fat whipped cream or yogurt

1. In a small bowl, whisk together balsamic vinegar, brown sugar, and pepper until combined.

2. Add berries, stir to combine, and let rest for 10 minutes.

3. Serve in dessert bowls, topped with whipped cream or yogurt.

Serves 4   PREP TIME: 15 MINUTES
PER SERVING: CALORIES: 44 FAT: 0.2 GRAM CHOLESTEROL: 0 MILLIGRAMS
SODIUM: 7.2 MILLIGRAMS CARBOHYDRATES: 10.7 GRAMS
FIBER: 2 GRAMS PROTEIN: 0.4 GRAM

Spiced Peaches with Ricotta

In the summer, when peaches are at their peak, try this simple but delicious preparation in place of more caloric desserts. Sucanat is the most commonly available brand of raw, unrefined cane sugar, which has its nutrients intact. It resembles cocoa powder. Other raw cane sugars or brown sugar will substitute well, but they won't be as healthy.

6 ripe peaches, pitted and thinly sliced
$\frac{1}{4}$ cup water
2 tablespoons Sucanat, or other raw or brown sugar
$1\frac{1}{2}$ tablespoons lemon juice
1 cup low-fat ricotta
2 teaspoons lemon zest

1. In a heavy, medium-sized skillet, combine peaches, water, Sucanat, and lemon juice. Bring just to a simmer, stirring frequently. Remove from heat.

2. In a small bowl, combine ricotta and lemon zest. Mix well.

3. Divide peaches between four bowls. Top with ricotta and serve.

Serves 4   PREP TIME: 15 MINUTES / COOKING TIME: 5 MINUTES
PER SERVING: CALORIES: 165 FAT: 5.2 GRAMS CHOLESTEROL: 19.1 MILLIGRAMS
SODIUM: 59 MILLIGRAMS CARBOHYDRATES: 25.6 GRAMS
FIBER: 2.9 GRAMS PROTEIN: 8 GRAMS

Fruited Oatmeal Cookies

These cookies get their moisture from yogurt and canola oil instead of butter. Dried fruit and dark chocolate chips make them seem like an indulgence, but they're actually cholesterol-free and full of healthful nutrients. A serving is one cookie.

1⅓ cups uncooked old-fashioned oats or quick-cooking rolled oats

1 cup whole-wheat flour

1 teaspoon baking powder

1 teaspoon ground cinnamon

¼ teaspoon ground mace

½ cup loosely packed brown sugar

⅓ cup plain low-fat yogurt

2 tablespoons canola oil

1 egg

1 teaspoon vanilla extract

½ cup mixed dried fruit

½ cup dark chocolate chips

1. Preheat oven to 350°F. Line two baking sheets with baking mats or parchment paper.

2. In a medium bowl, stir together oats, flour, baking powder, cinnamon, mace, and sugar.

3. In a large bowl, stir together yogurt, oil, egg, and vanilla. Add flour mixture to yogurt mixture. Using a spatula, mix until just combined. Stir in dried fruit and chocolate chips. ➤

Fruited Oatmeal Cookies *continued*

4. Using a tablespoon, drop cookie dough onto baking sheet about 2 inches apart.

5. Bake 10 to 12 minutes, until lightly browned. Remove from oven and cool on a wire rack.

———————

Makes 40 Cookies   PREP TIME: 10 MINUTES / COOKING TIME: 12 MINUTES
PER SERVING: CALORIES: 78 FAT: 3 GRAMS CHOLESTEROL: 0 MILLIGRAMS
SODIUM: 4 MILLIGRAMS CARBOHYDRATES: 12 GRAMS
FIBER: 2 GRAMS PROTEIN: 2 GRAMS

Ginger Molasses Cookies

These cookies are the DASH version of classic ginger spice cookies. Using minimal butter and an egg white instead of a whole egg reduces the cholesterol. A serving is one cookie.

3 tablespoons unsalted butter, softened
1 egg white
1 teaspoon vanilla extract
2 teaspoons blackstrap molasses
$3/4$ cup whole-wheat flour
$1/2$ cup all-purpose flour
$1/3$ cup granulated sugar
1 teaspoon baking soda
$1/2$ teaspoon ground ginger
$1/2$ teaspoon ground cinnamon
$1/4$ teaspoon ground nutmeg
1 teaspoon chopped crystallized ginger
Cooking spray

1. Preheat oven to 350°F.

2. In a large bowl, combine the butter, egg white, vanilla, and molasses. Mix until well blended.

3. In a medium bowl, whisk together the whole-wheat flour, all-purpose flour, sugar, baking soda, ground ginger, cinnamon, nutmeg, and crystallized ginger. ➤

Ginger Molasses Cookies *continued*

4. Add dry ingredients to wet ingredients, stirring until well mixed.

5. Using a tablespoon, drop dough 2 inches apart onto two baking sheets lightly coated with cooking spray. Bake for 15 minutes, or just until the cookies begin to brown on top and the edges.

6. Remove the baking sheets from the oven, and allow the cookies to sit on the sheets for 2 minutes before transferring them to a wire rack to cool.

Makes 40 Cookies   PREP TIME: 15 MINUTES / COOKING TIME: 15 MINUTES
PER SERVING: CALORIES: 61 FAT: 2 GRAMS CHOLESTEROL: 6 MILLIGRAMS
SODIUM: 44 MILLIGRAMS CARBOHYDRATES: 10 GRAMS
FIBER: 0 GRAMS PROTEIN: 1 GRAM

Lemony Angel Food Mini Cakes

Those little cake pans you've had your eye on at the housewares store are perfect to manage portion control, or use a cupcake pan instead. Serve with fresh fruit and a drizzle of Fudgy Sauce (recipe on page 165) or Lightened Whipped Cream (recipe on page 160). A serving is one mini cake.

1/2 cup plus 2 tablespoons powdered sugar
1/2 cup all-purpose white flour
6 egg whites
3/4 teaspoon cream of tartar
1 teaspoon lemon flavor or lemon extract
1/2 cup granulated sugar

1. Preheat oven to 350°F. Spray mini cake pans or 8 cups of a cupcake pan with cooking spray.

2. In a medium bowl, sift together the powdered sugar and the flour until it is very fine. Sift two or three times to ensure even consistency.

3. Using a stand mixer or hand held mixer on high speed, whip the egg whites, cream of tartar, and lemon flavor or extract until just combined, 1 to 2 minutes. Add the granulated sugar, 1 tablespoon at a time, until the egg whites form stiff peaks. Do not overwhip the eggs. ➤

Lemony Angel Food Mini Cakes *continued*

4. Using a spatula, slowly fold the flour mixture into the egg whites until just combined. Pour batter into prepared pans, stopping ½ inch before the rim.

5. Place cake pans on a baking sheet. Bake for 15 minutes. To check for doneness, gently push on the top of the cakes. If they spring back, they're ready. If not, bake for 2 to 5 more minutes until done.

6. Cool on a wire rack.

Makes 8 Mini Cakes   PREP TIME: 15 MINUTES / COOKING TIME: 15 MINUTES
PER SERVING: CALORIES: 120 FAT: 2 GRAMS CHOLESTEROL: 0 MILLIGRAMS
SODIUM: 1 MILLIGRAM CARBOHYDRATES: 22.6 GRAMS
FIBER: 0.5 GRAM PROTEIN: 5 GRAMS

Cinnamon Apple Cake

This bakes more quickly when you divide the batter among four 4½-inch mini-springform pans.

Cooking spray
1¾ cups granulated sugar
3 teaspoons ground cinnamon
1½ cups all-purpose flour
1½ teaspoons baking powder
½ teaspoon ground ginger
¼ teaspoon ground nutmeg
¼ teaspoon ground mace
½ cup (4 ounces) low-fat cream cheese
⅓ cup unsweetened applesauce
2 tablespoons canola oil
1 teaspoon vanilla extract
2 egg whites
3 Fuji apples, peeled and chopped into 1-inch pieces

1. Preheat oven to 350°F. Spray an 8-inch springform pan or four mini springform pans with cooking spray.

2. In a small bowl, mix ¼ cup of the sugar with 2 teaspoons of the cinnamon. Set aside.

3. In a medium bowl, combine flour, baking powder, ginger, nutmeg, mace, and remaining teaspoon cinnamon. Set aside. ➤

Cinnamon Apple Cake *continued*

4. In the bowl of a stand mixer fitted with the paddle attachment, beat 1½ cups sugar, cream cheese, applesauce, canola oil, and vanilla extract until well blended, about 4 minutes. Add egg whites to batter and continue beating until incorporated. Add flour mixture to batter, ¼ cup at a time, mixing until well incorporated.

5. In another small bowl, mix the apples with 3 tablespoons of the cinnamon sugar mixture. Gently stir the apple-cinnamon mixture into the batter.

6. Pour the batter into the pan or pans, and sprinkle with the remaining cinnamon sugar.

7. Bake for 20 minutes, or until a toothpick inserted in the center comes out clean. Individual pans will cook more quickly; check after 12 minutes.

Serves 16   PREP TIME: 15 MINUTES / COOKING TIME: 20 MINUTES
PER SERVING: CALORIES: 341 FAT: 12 GRAMS CHOLESTEROL: 62 MILLIGRAMS
SODIUM: 137 MILLIGRAMS CARBOHYDRATES: 57 GRAMS
FIBER: 3 GRAMS PROTEIN: 4 GRAMS

Don't get too upset if you take one step back. Holidays especially can challenge even a person with the willpower of Gandhi. Do your best in the situation, then review your journal and food triggers to see what you can change the next time. Change takes time. Your two steps forward are just around the corner.

Regard your DASH diet as an adventure. You are making a conscious choice to improve your health, and that means expanding your meal options, not limiting them. Try new recipes and foods that tantalize your taste buds rather than missing the foods you no longer include in your diet. Research interesting ingredients, and take some classes to expand your healthy cooking techniques and cuisines. Eating should nourish your body and your spirit, so enjoy the DASH experience.

Resources

The American Heart Association
www.heart.org
The website of the American Heart Association offers many tools, tips, and resources to keep you motivated.

DASH Diet Support Group
http://dashdiet.org/dash_support_group.asp
Joining an online or in-person support group is a great way to keep motivated and working toward your weight-loss goals.

Mydashdiet
http://appcrawlr.com/ios/mydashdiet

Calorie Counter Pro by Mynetdiary
http://appcrawlr.com/ios/calorie-counter-pro-by-mynetdia
These apps help you keep track of how much and what you eat using your mobile phone.

References

Davis, William, MD, *Wheat Belly*. New York: Rodale, 2011.

Bales, Connie, PhD, RD; Laura Svetkey, MD, MHS; Tamara Shusterman, MPH, RD; and Pao-Hwa Lin, PhD, *Eating Well, Living Well with Hypertension*. New York: Penguin Books, 1996.

Moore, Thomas, MD; Laura Svetkey, MD; Pao-Hwa Lin, PhD, and Njeri Karanja, PhD, with Mark Jenkins. *The DASH Diet for Hypertension*. New York: The Free Press, 2001.

Murty, C. M., J. K. Pittaway, and M. J. Ball. Chickpea supplementation in an Australian diet affects food choice, satiety, and bowel health. *Appetite*. April 2010, 54 (2): 282–8. Epub November 27, 2009. 2010.

Whitaker, Julian, MD, *Reversing Hypertension*. New York: Warner Books, 2000.

Recipe Index

Index

CPSIA information can be obtained
at www.ICGtesting.com
Printed in the USA
BVOW05s1437161116

468031BV00002B/15/P